KU-671-650

WE'D BE LOST WITHOUT BECKY and her delicious recipes!

Jade

I HAVE CHOICES!
For the first time I feel confident in finding recipes that I can cook and bake that are straightforward and delicious!

Samantha

Becky's recipes are a game changer! This book should be called **'HOW TO FEEL PART OF THE FAMILY AGAIN'**, or 'How to Actually Enjoy Food Again'. Just follow the recipes, you'll never look back!

Terrie

Makes cooking and eating gluten-free easy and tasty, **BECKY IS OUR SAVIOUR!**

Amy

Becky's recipes are **JUST WHAT THE GLUTEN-FREE COMMUNITY NEEDED**. To see that we can, and should be able to, eat anything again, with a few adaptations, is just so fantastic.

Debbie

'HOW IS THIS GLUTEN FREE?' Said my newly coeliac diagnosed 9-year-old! 'Becky is magic!'

Helena

Becky's recipes have never failed us. Every one we've tried has been amazing – gluten free food which tastes as good or often even better than muggle food! **I DON'T KNOW HOW SHE DOES IT**, but a massive thank you.

Karen and Tim

No fussy recipes just real down-to-earth delicious food. Your recipes make me and my daughter **FEEL NORMAL AGAIN!**

Laura

Becky's recipes are the easiest-to-follow gluten-free recipes I have ever seen, **NO FANCY FLOUR BLENDS**, just simple instructions using everyday ingredients.

Patricia

Becky's recipes are amazing because **I NEVER FEEL LIKE I'M MISSING OUT**, and I always trust that the end product will be amazing!

Katie

For all my lovely
followers who
have always
supported me and
trusted my recipes

How to

MAKE

anything

GLUTEN
FREE

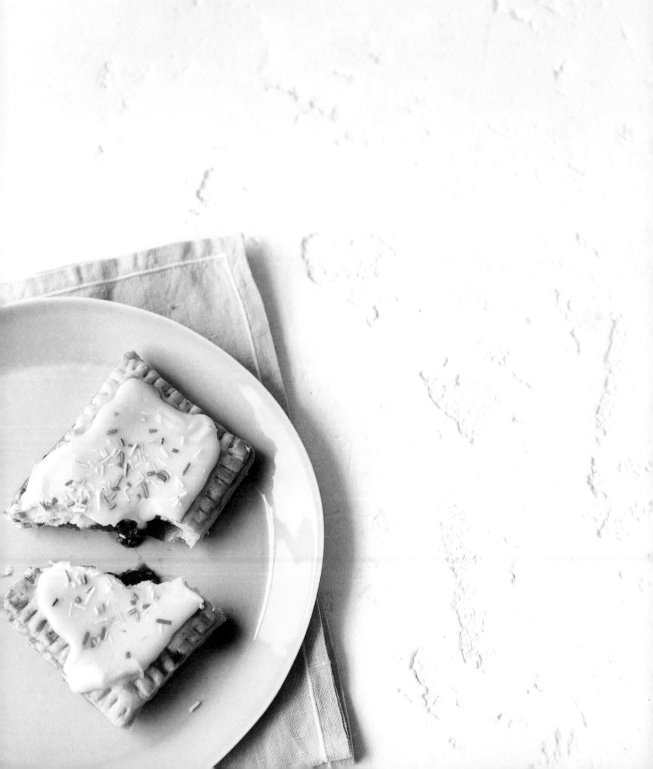

How to MAKE anything GLUTEN FREE

Over 100 Recipes for Everything
from Home Comforts to Fakeaways,
Cakes to Dessert, Brunch to Bread

BECKY EXCELL

Photography by Hannah Hughes

Hardie Grant

QUADRILLE

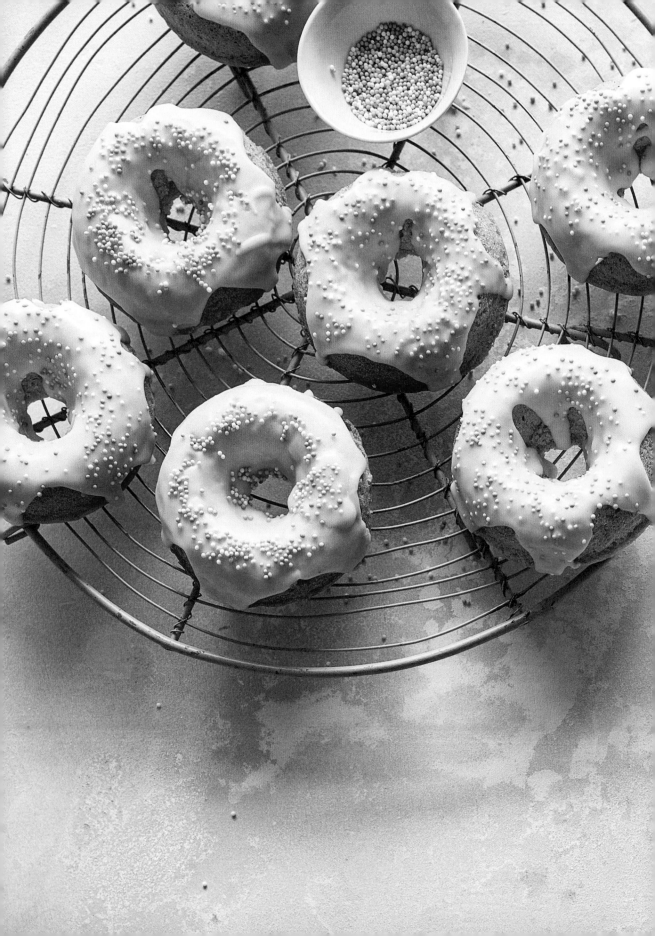

YOU'VE JUST OPENED THE BOOK THAT'LL SHOW YOU HOW TO UNLOCK ALL THE THINGS THAT YOU CAN NEVER ORDINARILY EAT ON A GLUTEN-FREE DIET. LET ME EXPLAIN...

Most people have a bucket list of things to do before they die. But not me. I have a bucket list of 100 things that I wish were gluten-free.

Sorry, I've just realized that I'm just literally listing foods that I can't eat. But, if you're gluten-free yourself (or you know someone who is) I bet you'll totally understand why I often get lost in my bucket list.

That's because, when you're gluten-free, all your favourite food instantly gets put on the list of things you **used** to eat. But do you forget about them and get on with your life?

OF COURSE NOT!

Instead, you gaze through the window of every bakery you pass, narrowly avoiding a head-on collision with a lamp post. You might occasionally catch yourself day-dreaming about when you last ate a **real** jam doughnut*. You're probably also filled with food envy whenever a fast-food ad comes on TV, uttering, 'I wish I could eat that' for the millionth time.

Being gluten-free made me realize that, when you're told you can't eat something, you only crave eating it ten times more. But there was one big problem with my gluten-free bucket list: I was probably never going to be able to eat any of the things on it ever again. After all, most things are utterly impossible to make gluten-free, right? And if they're not impossible, a 'gluten-free version' **always** tastes and/or looks worse – agreed?

Well, I've got a little news-flash for you that took me **years** to realize: it's not true. And I totally understand if you're filled with scepticism upon reading that. When I first became gluten-free twelve years ago (not sure why I've phrased that like I became a wizard at Hogwarts) I wouldn't have believed me either. But honestly, through years of travelling to gluten-free bakeries across the world and creating/sharing my own recipes online, I've discovered this:

YOU CAN MAKE ANYTHING GLUTEN-FREE

and even muggles* would never notice the difference.

Freshly baked bread, Chinese takeaway, fried jam doughnuts, homemade pastry, fresh pasta, classic cakes, bakery-style cookies, non-cardboard-tasting pizza...

It was 4,622 days ago FYI

people who can eat gluten

So, no – nothing needs to taste any different or look any worse either. Nor do you need tons of strange, unobtainable ingredients or a top-secret blend of gluten-free flour. I actually use a simple commercial gluten-free flour blend (if needed) for nearly every recipe in this book.

SO WHAT'S THE BIG SECRET, THEN?

Well, in the early years of being gluten-free, I'd naively try to replace wheat flour with gluten-free flour when following a recipe. Or even worse, I'd just skip those gluten-containing ingredients entirely.* Not surprisingly, I'd always end up wondering where it all went wrong and with a big mess to clear up.

*spoiler alert:

9 times out of 10, it just doesn't work.

And of course that didn't work! That's like reading a book, but removing the main character. Yes, you can still kind of follow the story, but the ending is probably going to be a big, confused mess. To truly get that happy ending, a gluten-free recipe needs to be its own unique story from start to finish.

THAT'S THE SECRET!

Oh, and just like on my blog, most of my recipes can easily be made dairy-free or lactose-free with simple swaps* and lots are easy to make vegan/veggie too. Plus, there are loads of recipes that are low FODMAP, which is handy if you suffer from IBS like I do.

*my boyfriend, Mark, is lactose intolerant and chief taste-tester, after all

So remember my bucket list of all the things I thought I'd never be able to eat again? Yep, I did it – I finally made them **all** gluten-free with zero compromise. And that's what you're holding right now – a collective list of all the things I once could only dream of eating. Now I can make them whenever I want, and so can you.

But if you still believe it's impossible to make anything gluten-free without compromise, that's OK. Because once you take a bite of something you haven't eaten in years **and** it tastes even better than you remember... you'll be so happy that you won't even mind me saying:

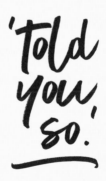

'told you, so.'

About me

I wish I could write this part in the third person so it didn't sound like I was tooting my own horn... Let's try it anyway. I'm Becky Excell, I've been gluten-free for over a decade and I share recipes online via my blog and on social media. I should probably also mention that 300,000+ people follow me and I won some awards and stuff too. That wasn't so painful to read, was it?

First of all, thanks for buying my debut cookbook, *How To Make Anything Gluten Free*. Or, if you're standing in a book shop considering buying it, then you definitely should because it's great (in my totally unbiased opinion).

Long story short – twelve years ago, my doctor diagnosed me with IBS and told me that my relationship with gluten was officially over. He probably should have tested me for coeliac disease before telling me not to eat gluten anymore, but I'm still working on my time machine to fix that part. Suddenly, I couldn't eat out anymore, I couldn't eat any of my favourite food and I was now confined to a tiny section of the supermarket. It was rubbish.

After a few years of eating tiny slices of gluten-free bread (which cost a small fortune) and watching my boyfriend eat 'real' pizza every week, I wasn't adjusting to gluten-free life well at all. Out of pure frustration, I got my apron on and began recreating all the things that I really missed eating. Then I'd post the recipes on my blog, just for safekeeping. But rather randomly, a handful of people started making my recipes, sending me photos of

their creations and thanking me. How on Earth did that happen?!

Fast-forward to today and that small handful of people has somehow turned into over a quarter of a million people. And I just want to take a second to thank each and every one of you who follows me. It goes without saying that this book wouldn't be possible without you – and that's why it is dedicated to all of you!

But even if you have no idea who I am at all, then great – I'm so glad you found this book anyway! I guess that if I had to sum up everything I do in one sentence, it would be this: I pride myself on creating recipes that show you how to unlock all the things that you could never ordinarily eat on a gluten-free diet. And I do that without using tons of hard-to-source ingredients or overly complex methods. I've just realized that was definitely two sentences. Oh and nobody would ever know that any of my creations were gluten-free either. Oops, that's three sentences now... this isn't going well at all, is it?

Did you notice the key distinction there, though? My recipes focus on unlocking all the things you *can't* normally eat on a gluten-free diet. Not the things you can. So no, this book isn't crammed full of recipes that are *naturally* gluten-free and never had gluten in them to start with. Oddly enough, it's hard to miss soups, salads and fruit when you can still eat them!

But if I'm allowed to toot my own horn once more, I think that small (but super important) distinction

is why people have grown to love my recipes. Ever since starting my blog, I've made it my mission to reunite people with their 'gluten-free bucket lists' by recreating all the things they can no longer eat. And in this book, I've tried to do that 100 times across 100 recipes.

So it goes without saying that I really hope you enjoy the journey of rediscovery that this recipe book will take you on. When I first had to go gluten-free over a decade ago, I wish I'd had a book like this. So I wrote it for all of you instead. And brief disclaimer: I'm certainly no professional chef, baker or scientist, so if I can create these recipes, then you definitely can too. Promise!

Don't forget that my recipes don't end with the last page of this book, either. Please go and check out my blog (glutenfreecuppatea.co.uk), Instagram or YouTube channel for tons more recipes and inspiration too. I'll be posting step-by-step video tutorials to accompany the recipes in this book over on my YouTube channel and featuring more photos of the dishes not pictured in this book on my blog (just search 'HTMAGF'). So definitely come over and say hi.

Most importantly, if you do try one of my recipes, please make sure you take a photo before you eat it (I know it's hard). Then, simply post it online and tag me in it – it absolutely makes my day seeing all of your creations!

Becky x

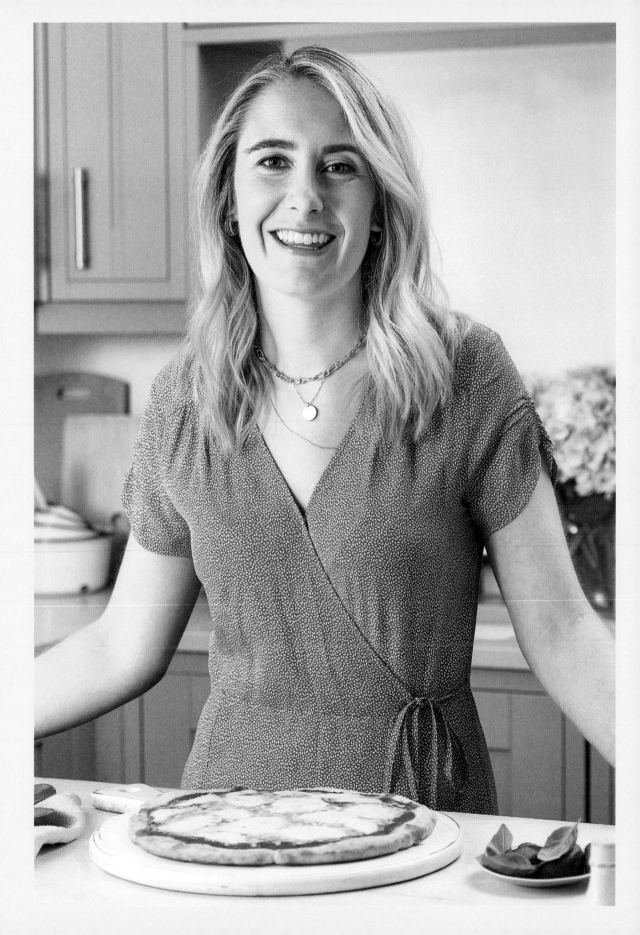

A crash-course in
PREPARING GLUTEN-FREE FOOD

If you're cooking for yourself or someone else who's gluten-free (lucky them!) there are three simple things you need to know to ensure that your wondrous creation is safe to eat. After all, even the tiniest amount of gluten can be harmful.

So when preparing gluten-free food, it's important to ask yourself these three questions:

1.
Do any of the ingredients or products have any gluten-containing ingredients or relevant allergen warnings?

First of all, triple-check the ingredients list on any products used to ensure that they don't have any gluten-containing ingredients or relevant 'may contain' allergy warnings. Here's a list of common sources of gluten that you'll need to avoid:

- wheat
- barley
- rye
- oats (see page 12 for more on oats)
- spelt

Of course, even if a product doesn't have any gluten-containing ingredients, it can still be cross-contaminated through manufacturing methods.

Even naturally gluten-free products like beansprouts or hazelnuts can sometimes have 'may contain' warnings that makes them unsuitable for most people who are gluten-free. I've even seen 'may contain' warnings on salt and pepper, so it's best to check everything.

I've indicated each ingredient in this book as 'gluten-free' where commonly necessary. But it's still best to triple check the ingredients and allergy info on the packaging of every product you're using.

2.
How can I store my ingredients or products separately from gluten-containing foods?

If a gluten-free product or ingredient comes into contact with gluten at any point, it's no longer truly gluten-free. So how can you minimize that risk? Here are a few common best practices:

- Firstly, once gluten-free products are removed from their packaging, they must immediately be stored separately from gluten-containing products. This can easily be achieved by using sealed, airtight containers. It's also wise to label the containers so it's clear to everyone in the household what's inside.

- Also, remember: if you butter gluten bread, then put the knife back into the butter, the butter is no longer gluten-free. It's always a good idea to have separate butter/jam/peanut butter and condiments that are clearly labelled as being 'gluten-free only'.

3.
How can I avoid cross-contamination when preparing and cooking gluten-free food?

Carefully considering your cooking methods and any equipment used is vital in preparing gluten-free food, especially if your kitchen or utensils have previously been used to prepare gluten-containing food.

So how can you minimize that risk? Here's a few more best practices:

- Of course, gluten-free food must be cooked *entirely* separately from gluten-containing food.

- When deep-frying gluten-free food, do not reuse oil that has been previously used to cook gluten-containing food.

- Do not place gluten-free bread in a toaster that has been used for gluten-containing bread.

- Do not cut gluten-free bread on a board that has been used for gluten-containing bread.

- All utensils and surfaces must be cleaned if they have previously come into contact with gluten. You can happily use washing-up liquid and dishwashers to do this.

- Ideally, you'd own utensils, pans and bread boards that are solely dedicated to gluten-free cooking.

The moral of the story is that you can never be too careful! This isn't an exhaustive list, so definitely visit the website of your country's coeliac society for up-to-date info.

Gluten-free
STORE-CUPBOARD INGREDIENTS

As I said in the introduction of this book, a gluten-free recipe absolutely must be its own unique story. So allow me to introduce all the 'characters' you'll meet across this book to ensure that it has a happy ending!

I've endeavoured to ensure that over 90% of these ingredients are easily sourced in supermarkets. But you may have to hop online for two of the 'wonder' ingredients that I use in the bread chapter – trust me, it's worth it for fresh bread that tastes like real fresh bread!

This isn't an exhaustive list of every gluten-free flour out there (there are tons more!), just the ones I use in this book.

FLOUR

Gluten-free plain (all-purpose) flour

So often when I state 'gluten-free plain flour' on my blog, some people take it as meaning a *singular* type of gluten-free flour. For example: coconut flour or buckwheat flour. But gluten-free plain (or all-purpose) flour refers to a *blend* of different gluten-free flours. The gluten-free plain flour I use in this book is Freee (Doves Farm) and can be easily found in supermarkets in the UK. It is a blend of rice, potato, tapioca, maize and buckwheat flour – look for something similar in whichever country you live.

Due to the nature of being 'plain', it has no added xanthan gum (read on to find out what on Earth it even is) and no added raising agents. If you can't find a decent gluten-free plain flour where you live, there's a blend on my blog that you can easily make in no time at all.

Gluten-free self-raising (self-rising) flour

So here's the non 'plain' version of gluten-free flour which commonly has a little added xanthan gum and raising agents too. This flour is essentially used whenever you're looking for a nice rise in your baking, though it's not totally uncommon to still add a little extra baking powder for good measure. If you can't find gluten-free self-raising flour where you live, use the simple recipe on page 36 to make your own from a plain (all-purpose) blend.

Gluten-free white bread flour

Gluten-containing bread flour is extremely high in gluten, which makes it ideal for baking bread. Gluten-free bread flour obviously isn't quite as magical and you'll still need psyllium husk (read more about it on page 14) to compensate for the lack of gluten when baking bread. But nevertheless, it still gets the job done! Mine contains rice flour, potato starch, tapioca starch and xanthan gum but, in a pinch, you can substitute it for gluten-free plain flour. This is another one that I simply buy in the supermarket.

Cornflour (cornstarch)

This amazing starch is key to so many of my best gluten-free recipes. Not to be confused with maize flour or cornmeal, cornflour is a starch that's often used to thicken sauce and gravy. It's readily available in supermarkets, hence why I prefer to use it over other harder-to-source gluten-free starches. It makes any batter much lighter and puffier, it's the key to my huge Yorkshire puddings, and adding it to my fried doughnuts or cookies gives them a perfect texture.

Gluten-free buckwheat flour

Despite having a curse word in the name (wheat), buckwheat flour is actually derived from fruit seeds. That makes it naturally gluten-free, but watch out for 'may contain' warnings on the packaging as it can often be cross-contaminated during manufacturing too. This flour has tons of wholegrain flavour, which is perfect in my artisan loaf (page 42) and makes awesome French galettes (page 74).

Gram (garbanzo bean) flour

Alternatively known as chickpea flour or besan flour, this flour is (not surprisingly) made from chickpeas. That means that it's high in protein and has a yellow hue to it. Since gluten is a protein and we're always eliminating it from recipes, adding a source of protein helps massively when you're working with dough. Look out for it in the 'international' section of the supermarket. While naturally gluten-free, watch out for 'may contain' warnings on the packaging as it can also often be cross-contaminated during manufacturing.

Rice flour

While buckwheat flour adds a wholegrain-like taste, rice flour comes with a more neutral flavour. That's why it works perfectly in my gluten-free white sandwich loaf (page 41). It has a high starch content that can help with elasticity, which is very helpful when you're baking without gluten.

Masa harina flour

This is a special type of treated maize flour used in Latin America. The cooked kernels are nixtamalized by soaking them in lime water, then ground into masa harina flour, which is gluten-free. I use it to make authentic Mexican corn tortilla wraps which are naturally gluten-free (page 59). You can easily find it online; just ensure it's clearly labelled as 'masa harina flour' or states 'harina de maíz nixtamalizado' on the packaging. Don't use regular cornflour or cornmeal instead of masa harina flour – it won't work!

Pre-cooked cornmeal flour

Though also derived from corn, this naturally gluten-free flour is sometimes also known as 'masarepa flour' and is very different to cornflour and masa harina. Not surprisingly, it's predominantly used to make arepas (page 60), a South American corn cake that you can pack lots of savoury fillings into. Unlike regular cornmeal, this has already been cooked, and that makes a big difference. So definitely don't use regular cornmeal in place of this either, it must be pre-cooked. You can easily find it online.

SIMPLE SWAPS

Gluten-free oats

While oats are naturally gluten-free, unless they're labelled as 'gluten-free oats', regular oats will be cross-contaminated through production methods. In fact, in some countries, oats are never truly considered to be gluten-free. A small number of people still struggle to tolerate oats, despite them being totally gluten-free, so do be aware of that.

Gluten-free baking powder

Baking powder is one of those tricky ingredients that isn't actually always gluten-free. Some brands of baking powder often add wheat flour to their baking powder to help bulk it out or absorb water. Not only does that mean it's no longer gluten-free, but having wheat in baking powder also makes it worse as a raising agent! Just be sure to always check the label.

Gluten-free soy sauce (tamari)

This magic liquid is a no-brainer for recreating fakeaway meals at home, and instantly adds a lovely umami flavour. Sometimes I even take a bottle with me if I'm eating out – fortunately, it hasn't leaked yet! As you can't currently buy gluten-free dark soy sauce anywhere on Earth, check page 35 to see how to make your own using three simple ingredients.

Gluten-free dried pasta

I almost wrote 'dried gluten-free pasta isn't that bad' before realizing that made it sound way worse than it actually is. Taste and texture wise, it's actually great but when cooking, it gets slightly sticky and can clump together when boiled. But you can easily combat this by adding a little oil and salt to the pasta water. Of course, you can always make your own fresh gluten-free pasta using the recipe on page 24.

Gluten-free breadcrumbs

While you can always make your own using the recipe on page 32, buying some ready-made gluten-free breadcrumbs can be a massive timesaver. You can use them to quickly coat chicken in breadcrumbs for my katsu curry on page 113, or use them to make my homemade Scotch eggs (page 96).

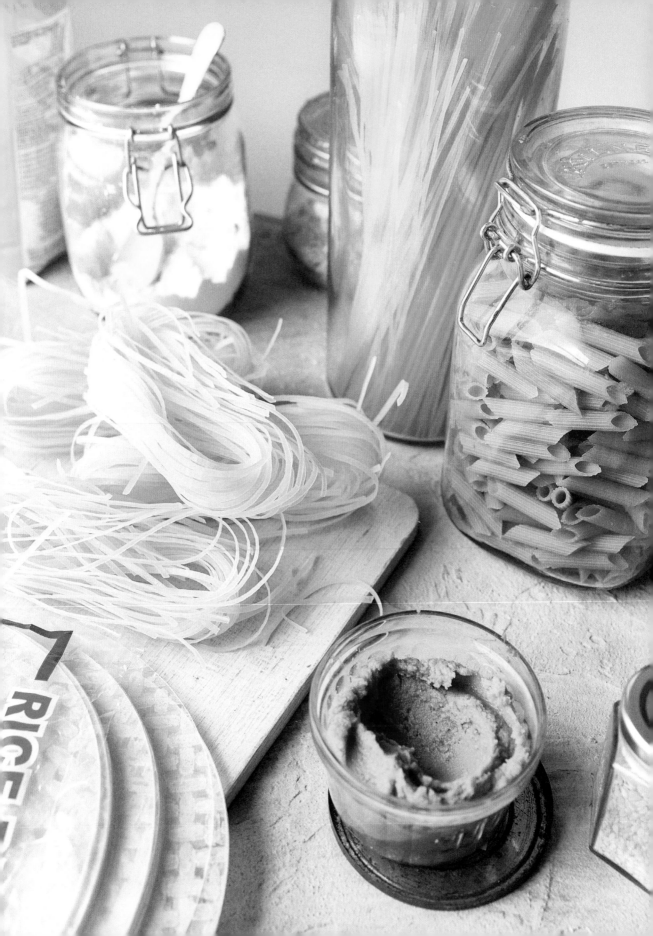

Gluten-free stock cubes

Fortunately for us, there seems to be a wide variety of gluten-free stock cubes out there in supermarkets at the moment. Most of them are clearly labelled as 'gluten-free' and having a good supply in the cupboard at home is never a bad thing. You can also now find gluten-free and low FODMAP stock cubes online.

Dry sherry

This is an amazing substitute for Shaoxing rice wine, which is a traditional Chinese wine used in lots of authentic recipes – the only problem? It contains wheat! However, dry sherry has a similar flavour and is a perfect like-for-like replacement. You'll need this in a few of my fakeaway recipes and in my auntie's trifle recipe (page 212) too.

Gluten-free Worcestershire sauce

Worcestershire sauce is a condiment that you can easily find a gluten-free substitute for in the supermarket. While this is an optional ingredient for this recipe book, you never know when you might need an instant injection of flavour.

Rice noodles

I'm sure that everyone who's gluten-free is more than familiar with rice noodles by now – that's all we're ever allowed to eat! These are naturally gluten-free and often come as either vermicelli or flat ribbon noodles. I find that dried rice noodles which also have a little tapioca starch in them to be the best by far. They have more of a bite to them and don't break anywhere near as easily when stir-frying. Of course, you can always make your own gluten-free egg noodles using the recipe on page 34.

Rice paper spring roll wrappers

These are commonly used in Vietnamese cooking to make summer rolls – a non-deep-fried cousin of the spring roll. They're often made purely from rice and tapioca flour, so they're naturally gluten-free unless otherwise stated. I tend to find them in the supermarket with all the Chinese-style sauces and condiments and use them to make summer rolls, then deep-fry them to make quick and easy gluten-free spring rolls (page 81).

BINDING

Xanthan gum

This should be a staple ingredient in every gluten-free person's cupboard. But with a name like that, what even is it? Well, it's used in food products as a thickener or stabilizer thanks to its binding properties. But in gluten-free food, it's effectively used as a replacement for gluten's natural elasticity. In gluten-free cakes and bread, it stops the consistency from being loose, crumbly and brittle, and a little goes a long way. It comes in a powder form and can be found in your supermarket's gluten-free aisle. It's not the end of the world if you don't use it BUT it definitely helps, especially in bread!

Psyllium husk powder

I wanted to make sure that this book wasn't crammed full of unusual ingredients, but this one is so integral to baking gluten-free bread that I absolutely had to include it. In case you're wondering, psyllium husk is a form of dietary fibre made from the seeds of a *Plantago* plant.

It works in a similar way to xanthan gum as a gluten replacer but it provides a 'bread-like' texture that xanthan gum can't match. When buying it online, firstly make sure it's psyllium husk *powder* as you can also buy a non-powdered version. But most importantly, please ensure it's clearly labelled as gluten-free as some can have a 'may contain' warning on them. It's a must-have ingredient for gluten-free bread bakers!

Other handy

INGREDIENTS

Here are all the everyday ingredients used throughout this book. While they should all be naturally gluten-free, it doesn't hurt to double-check the label just in case.

Active dried yeast

This is the only type of yeast I'll be using in this book. Active dried yeast needs to be dissolved in a warm liquid and activated prior to using. But don't fret – you'll see this reflected in the recipe method where necessary. Yeast isn't always gluten-free as other ingredients may be added, so ensure that yours is safe before using. Oh, and make sure that your yeast isn't out of date, otherwise it won't work!

Eggs

Where necessary, I've indicated throughout this book whether you'll need small, medium or large eggs. It can make a big difference, especially in baking! But, did you know that a large egg in the UK is actually bigger than in the USA, Canada and Australia? Because of this, I've included a handy egg 'conversion' guide at the back of this book on page 216. This will be useful if you're from one of the above locations. PS. If so, can I please come and visit?

Butter

I've always used margarine in my cakes since I can remember. It's what my mum used and it's what my grandma always used too. But if you can tolerate dairy products, I've come to realize that you simply can't beat a real block of butter for gluten-free baking; it's not just for flavour – its high fat content makes any dough much more workable. That's especially important when you're baking without gluten.

Hard dairy-free butter alternative

When making a recipe dairy-free, my go-to replacement for butter has always been a block of hard margarine (also known as a baking block). Unlike margarine that you'd spread on toast, this margarine comes in a hard block. It's much better at replacing butter in things like cookies or pastry, where soft, spreadable margarine just wouldn't work. Despite being a hard block, it's still softer than butter, so bear that in mind when making pastry or icing. Even if you can't find a hard block of margarine where you live, any hard block of vegan butter works well too – just ensure it's completely dairy-free with no 'may contain' warnings.

Dairy-free milk

Of course, if you're dairy-free, you can always substitute milk with whatever dairy-free milk you'd prefer. Results can vary depending on which type of milk you're using. For example, I usually find that pancakes often come out looking paler as a result of using dairy-free milk, so bear that in mind!

Lactose-free milk

My boyfriend is lactose intolerant, so we always have lactose-free milk in the fridge. Lactose-free milk is *real* cow's milk, but with an enzyme called 'lactase' added to help cancel out the lactose. Using real milk or lactose-free milk has absolutely no impact on a recipe, so feel free to use them interchangeably if you need to.

Greek yoghurt

You might be surprised to find that Greek yoghurt is a staple ingredient when I make any kind of gluten-free flatbread or pizza. It's lovely and thick and full of protein, which binds together wonderfully with a gluten-free flour blend. You can now commonly find lactose-free Greek yoghurt in supermarkets.

Black treacle

Black treacle is basically the British version of molasses. So if you can't find it, feel free to substitute it like-for-like if needed.

Golden syrup

This is yet another British store-cupboard staple, sometimes known as light or golden treacle. It's essentially a form of inverted sugar syrup with a distinctive 'buttery' taste. Here in the UK you'll find it with all the other syrups in the supermarket, but it seems to be available all across the world these days – check the international aisle of your supermarket. Trust me, it's worth hunting for!

Garlic-infused oil

This is the ultimate must-have ingredient in our house. First of all, this will save you tons of time on peeling, chopping and cooking garlic. It's an instant injection of wonderful garlic flavour and, if you're intolerant to garlic like I am, then it's even more invaluable. That's because as long as it doesn't have any visible bits of garlic floating in it, garlic-infused oil is low FODMAP and suitable for those who can't tolerate garlic. You'll find it in your supermarket's cooking oil aisle.

Miso paste

Mark and I endeavoured to make all of our gluten-free Chinese fakeaway recipes as authentic as possible. But where we couldn't find easily accessible ingredients like fermented yellow bean paste or 'meju' (fermented soybeans) for my Korean-style chilli sauce, we discovered that miso paste does a very similar job - it's made from fermented soybeans after all! Most are gluten-free, but not all. So, double-check the ingredients and 'may contain' allergy warnings first.

Fresh chives

If you've ever watched my YouTube videos, you'll likely know that the final thing I'll say when making dinner is 'and then sprinkle on some fresh, chopped chives'. Why? Well, chives add an instant, onion flavour that perfectly finishes off any savoury dish. They are also a godsend when you can't tolerate onion!

Spring onions (scallions)

The same goes for spring onions too - simply chop and throw onto any savoury dish for a lovely, fresh, slightly more intense onion flavour. If you're low FODMAP or intolerant to onion, then ensure that you only eat the green parts at the top.

Minced ginger paste

Minced ginger is one of those magic ingredients that can save you tons of time when you're cooking. Feel free to buy that big hunk of fresh ginger if you like, but I promise that your life will be changed by keeping a little jar of minced ginger in the fridge. It's ready to add - no chopping required. You can usually find it with all the other spices in the supermarket.

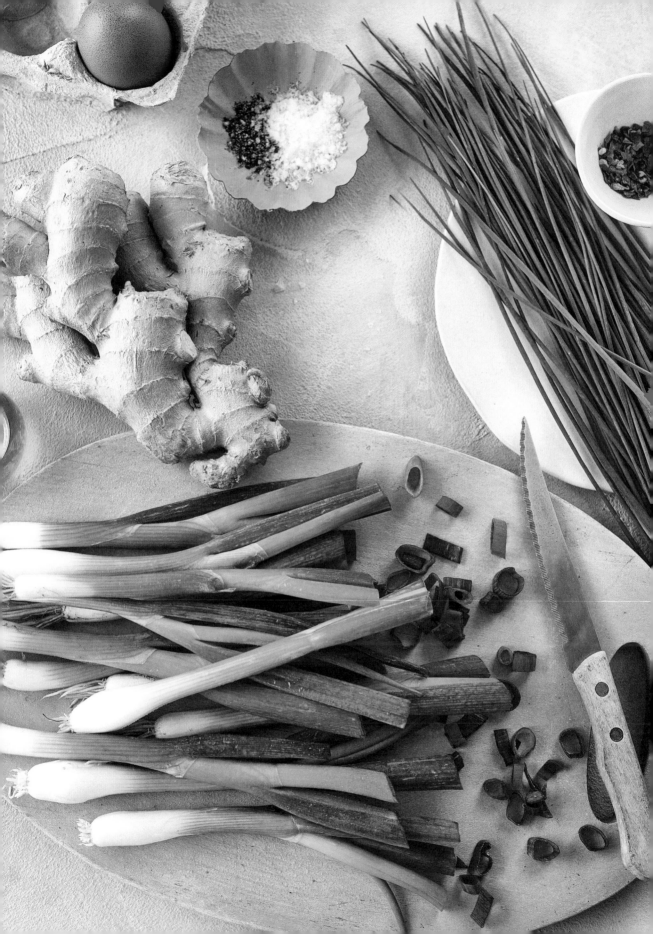

Useful
EQUIPMENT

These are what I'd class as the essentials for cooking and baking, assuming you have a decent set of sharp knives, pots, pans and a few baking trays already. While not everything is mandatory for this book, if you do have everything listed here then you can basically create anything!

Fan oven

Obviously, having *any* kind of oven helps massively when you're baking! But I included this here mainly to emphasize that all the recipes in this book were developed using a fan oven. I've given non-fan and Fahrenheit temperatures too, so just use those if you don't use a fan oven.

Digital weighing scales

I can't emphasize how important it is to weigh out your ingredients with digital cooking scales for gluten-free baking. The difference of 10 grams or millilitres can make a huge difference between a workable dough and a wet, sticky dough: unlike baking with gluten, gluten-free baking has very little margin for error.

12-hole muffin or cupcake tray

I'd struggle to count the number of different things I've used a humble muffin tray for throughout this book. There's everything from pork pies to Yorkshire puddings, cupcakes, muffins, pastéis de nata and beyond. Invest in a good, heavy-duty muffin tray and thank me later.

20cm / 8in round baking tins (pans)

I'd recommend getting two (or maybe even three) of these for baking. That's because you often make two or three sponges for a full cake and baking them all separately not only takes ages, but the cake batter can begin to dry out – this usually means it won't rise well as a result.

20cm / 8in round loose-bottomed baking tins (pans)

Either loose-bottomed or springform baking tins are perfect for making the cheesecakes in this book. I personally prefer loose-bottomed over springform as I find it much easier to get my cheesecake off the base after, but both work well. Also, these tend to have much higher sides than regular round baking tins.

23cm / 9in square baking tin (pan)

The number of things you can make in a humble square baking tin never ceases to blow my mind. Think brownies, focaccia and breakfast bars. Plus, when you slice your creation up, you'll get perfectly square, equal slices, which you don't get with a round baking tin.

23cm / 9in fluted tart tin (pan)

For baking anything from a quiche to a lemon tart, a fluted tart tin gives you that perfect pastry case shape. Mine is also loose bottomed, which makes removing the tart an infinitely less stressful process.

900g / 2lb loaf tin (pan)

For all of my gluten-free loaf cakes, you'll need a 900g (2lb) loaf tin to get the job done. You don't need to break the bank for one of these, as even the cheapest options seem to be pretty durable.

25cm / 10in bread tin (pan)

Unless you like your gluten-free bread to be fun-sized, investing in a decent sized bread tin is always a good idea. Mine is 26 x 12 x 8cm (10 x 4¾ x 3¼in) in size.

Baguette tray

This is my prized possession. Why? Well, these relatively inexpensive yet invaluable trays are the only way to create lovely, long sticks of gluten-free French bread. Mine is 39 x 16.5 x 2.5cm (15¼ x 6½ x 1in) in size.

Proving basket (banneton)

If you fancy making my gluten-free soda bread or artisan loaf, you'll need one of these to prove it in. It ensures that the dough proves into a lovely boule shape, which you can then turn out into a skillet or ovenproof dish. Mine is 22cm (8½in) in diameter. Failing that you can always use a bowl lined with a clean tea (dish) towel.

28cm and 20cm / 11in and 8in skillets

I had no idea what I'd use a skillet, (or ovenproof frying pan) for when I bought one, but I seem to find more and more uses for it every day. In this book I use an 11in skillet to bake my soda bread, artisan loaf, gnocchi bake and mac and cheese. I use my 8in skillet for my triple cheese doughballs and gooey skillet cookie. Of course, they're not mandatory for this book, or those recipes, but they certainly make life a lot easier instead of trying to use a rectangular ovenproof dish for everything!

Rolling pin

If you intend to venture into baking gluten-free pastry, pasta or flatbreads, then a good rolling pin will definitely be your friend. Mine comes with a variety of thickness ring guides that assist you in rolling your dough out to a specific thickness - utterly invaluable!

Sieve

Not only is a sieve integral to tons of the baking recipes in this book, but there's another very important reason that I mention it here. Please make sure your sieve hasn't previously been used to sift wheat flour without being properly cleaned! Also, consider labelling it so anyone else in your house knows it's for gluten-free flour only.

Non-stick baking parchment

I've learned the hard way that there are definitely different grades of non-stick baking parchment. The cheapest grade still sticks and the more expensive brands are *actually* non-stick! So this might be an area that's worth investing in as you'll need it a lot for baking.

Wok

For tons of the fakeaway recipes in this book, you'll need a good-quality, non-stick wok. It doesn't have to be the biggest in the world, but it would help!

Stand mixer

While you can always achieve the same results that a stand mixer can simply by using a mixing bowl and a spatula, it'll probably take you triple the time. When it comes to mixing buttercream or especially when whisking meringue, I always let my stand mixer do all of the hard work for me.

Food processor

The same goes for a food processor. I use mine to blitz biscuits for the base of a cheesecake, blend prawns for prawn toast and to make my own gluten-free breadcrumbs out of stale bread. It makes the job so quick and, needless to say, it's so handy to have when you need it.

Electric hand whisk

Before I was able to afford a stand mixer, I used an electric hand whisk for nearly all mixing. So if you don't have a stand mixer, this can be a much cheaper option for mixing up icing and cake batter.

Digital cooking thermometer

I can't emphasize enough how much easier your cooking life could be if you owned a digital cooking thermometer. Not only can you use it to make sure meat is cooked before cutting into it, but it's great for whenever you're deep-frying food too. Instead of guessing when the oil is hot enough, you'll know exactly when it's ready to fry.

Wooden spoon

You might be surprised to learn that I very rarely use a wooden spoon when I'm baking (I use a silicone spatula for that). Instead, I use my humble wooden spoon to check the temperature of my oil for deep frying. Simply pop the handle into the oil for 3-4 seconds - if you see bubbles gently forming around it then it's ready to fry. The wooden spoon handle test has never let me down yet!

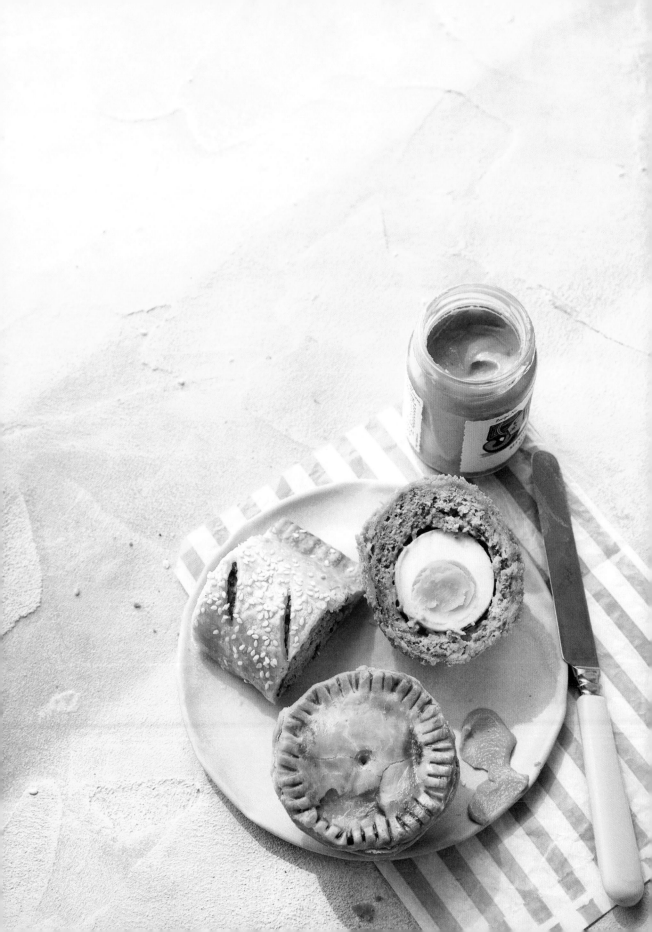

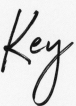

Key

Of course, everything in this entire book is gluten-free! But I've also labelled all of my recipes to clearly indicate whether they're dairy-free, lactose-free, low lactose, vegetarian, vegan or low FODMAP. But even if a recipe isn't naturally suitable for all dietary requirements, watch out for the little additional helpful notes by the key. These will indicate any simple swaps you can implement in order to adapt that recipe to your dietary requirements, if possible.

Also, if the recipe needs more than a couple of simple tweaks, make sure you check the 'Making it...?' section underneath each recipe for full advice on how to adapt it.

Here's a breakdown of what labels I'll be using so you know what they look like and exactly what I mean when I use them.

Vegetarian

This indicates that a recipe is meat- and fish-free. Recently, we have been trying to juggle eating more vegetarian meals alongside our other intolerances – so far, so good! Though most savoury dishes in this book require a little adapting to make them veggie, I've added simple suggestions throughout on how we make them meat-free at home. Make sure all products and ingredients used are vegetarian-friendly.

Vegan

This indicates that a recipe contains no ingredients that are derived from animals. Even if a recipe isn't vegan to start with, look out for my helpful notes for simple swaps, or check the 'Making it...?' section at the bottom of each recipe. If it is possible to make the recipe using alternatives to meat, eggs, etc., I'll tell you how. Make sure all products and ingredients used are vegan-friendly.

Dairy-free

This indicates that a recipe contains zero dairy products. Ensure no ingredient has a 'may contain' warning for traces of dairy and double-check that everything used is 100% dairy-free. Also, fun fact: eggs are *not* a dairy product. As one of my followers once said: 'When's the last time you saw a cow lay an egg?' They had a good point! If a recipe calls for a quantity of one of my pastry recipes or pizza dough, ensure you make that dairy-free too.

Lactose-free

Lactose-free? Isn't that the same as dairy-free? No, it definitely isn't! For example, lactose-free milk is *real* cow's milk (see page 15), so while it's definitely not dairy-free, it is suitable for those with a lactose intolerance. The 'lactose-free' label indicates that a recipe is naturally lactose-free or uses lactose-free products.

Low lactose

Fun fact: a lot of hard cheese is so naturally low in lactose that people with a lactose intolerance will have no problems tolerating it in moderation. In case you didn't know, butter and most hard cheese (such as Parmesan, Cheddar, pecorino) are naturally low in lactose. That means you don't need to buy a special lactose-free version, unless you're eating large quantities of it. Of course, recipes that use these ingredients aren't technically lactose-free, so they'll be labelled as low lactose for clarity.

Low FODMAP

This indicates that one serving of the finished recipe is low FODMAP. The low FODMAP diet was specifically created by Monash University in order to help relieve the symptoms of IBS in sufferers. Brief disclaimer: you should always start the low FODMAP diet in consultation with your dietician.

Also, you might be surprised to find that there's no actual onion or garlic in any of the recipes in the book. Why? Well, they are two ingredients that most people with IBS can't tolerate – myself included! If you're in the same boat, please ensure that any products you cook with are low FODMAP. Here are a few quick side notes: whenever I mention spring onions in this book, I mean the green parts only for FODMAP reasons. Also, garlic-infused oil is low FODMAP as long as it's clear and doesn't visibly have bits of garlic floating in it.

Essentials

I thought it was pretty ironic that this chapter is called 'essentials' yet us gluten-free folks often go without everything I've included here. Apparently they're essential for everyone else, apart from us! Well, that changes now.

Here are all the recipes you'll need to make anything from rough puff pastry to pasta, dark soy sauce and even egg noodles, all from scratch and gluten-free.

I refer back to these recipes throughout the book a lot, so you definitely won't be short of ideas on how to use them. Of course, where store-bought options are available (like for pasta, breadcrumbs and shortcrust pastry) you can always use those for convenience too.

But, trust me, nothing is as good or as satisfying as making it yourself and showing gluten who's boss.

Fresh
PASTA

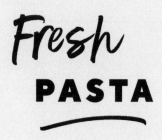

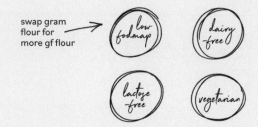

swap gram flour for more gf flour

low fodmap

dairy free

lactose free

vegetarian

MAKES · 500G / 18OZ COOKED PASTA (450G / 1LB UNCOOKED)

TAKES · 45 MINUTES

- 230g / 1⅔ cups gluten-free plain (all-purpose) flour, plus extra for dusting
- 50g / ⅖ cup gram (chickpea) flour
- 1 tsp xanthan gum
- 3 large eggs

While you can happily use dried gluten-free pasta from supermarkets throughout this book, there's something so satisfying about making your own from scratch. You can easily use this dough to make lasagne sheets and tagliatelle - and it's pasta machine friendly too!

In a large mixing bowl, mix together the flour, gram flour and xanthan gum, then make a well in the middle of the flour. Add the eggs and mix with a fork until all the egg is incorporated. Use your hands to form a slightly sticky dough ball.

Dough too wet and sloppy? Gradually add a teaspoon of extra flour until sticky. Dough too dry to form a ball? Gradually add a teaspoon of water.

On a well-floured surface, knead your dough for 1 minute or until it becomes smooth and no longer sticky. Place the dough ball back in the bowl and cover with cling film (plastic wrap). Allow to rest for 30 minutes – don't rush this part, it gives the dough much needed elasticity.

Cut the dough into equal quarters and take one portion of the dough, leaving the rest covered in the bowl so they don't dry out. From this point onwards, use as little flour as possible to dust your work surface and rolling pin - only add a little when the dough is sticking.

Using a rolling pin, roll out the dough on a *lightly* floured surface to a 5mm / ¼in thickness – aim for a long lasagne sheet shape. Fold in half like a book then fold over in half once more (the folding gives the dough strength and structure).

Roll the dough for a final time to a long lasagne sheet shape, this time aiming for a 1mm / ¹⁄₃₂in thickness so that it's paper thin and almost see-through. The pasta will double in thickness once cooked, so it's key to get it as thin as possible.

At this point, you could simply use a pizza cutter to cut out ready-to-use lasagne sheets, or keep following the instructions to make tagliatelle-style pasta.

Lightly flour the surface of your dough and rub it in so that the flour basically disappears. Very loosely fold over the bottom of the dough so that it meets the centre. Then loosely fold the top of the rolled-out dough over that. It should be folded up like a letter in an envelope with a little slack on each fold.

Take a long, sharp knife and trim off the untidy edges. Then smoothly cut the dough into 2-3mm / ¹⁄₁₆-⅛in strips; don't 'saw' the dough when cutting as it may tear, and take your time so that they're all a uniform size. Gently unravel your folded strips to reveal nice, long strips of dough. Place onto your lightly floured surface to avoid them sticking together.

Repeat the rolling and cutting with the rest of your dough.

To cook the pasta

Add half of your pasta to a large saucepan of boiling water with 1 tablespoon of salt added and cook for 4–5 minutes, then drain. Repeat with the other half of pasta then serve immediately with your chosen sauce. The pasta will likely be a little sticky, but the extra starch will disappear and magically thicken your sauce.

To create dried pasta

Once you've cut all your strips of tagliatelle, create four nests and allow to dry out for 24 hours on a wooden board, turning them over halfway. You can keep the dried pasta nests in an airtight container in the fridge for up to 5 days. Cook for 5-7 minutes.

TIP:
The less flour you use for dusting your rolling pin and work surfaces, the better. It can make your cooked pasta unpleasantly sticky and starchy.

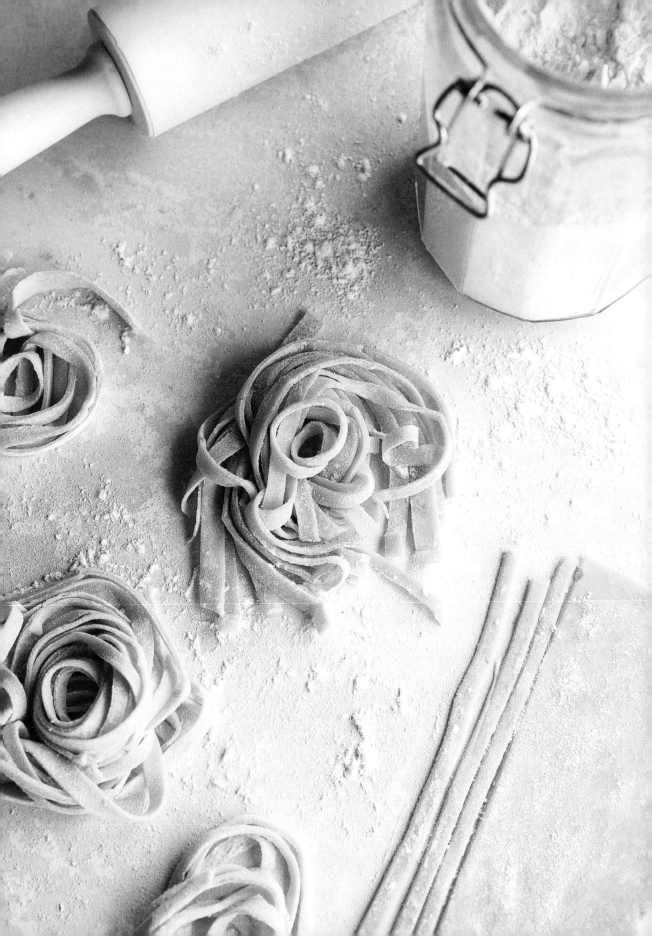

3-INGREDIENT
Potato Gnocchi

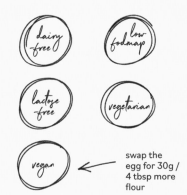

dairy free

low fodmap

lactose free

vegetarian

vegan

← swap the egg for 30g / 4 tbsp more flour

SERVES · 2-3 (MAKES 500G / 18OZ COOKED GNOCCHI OR 430G / 15OZ UNCOOKED)

TAKES · 1 HOUR

- 500g / 18oz potatoes, ideally Maris Piper (russet) or King Edward, scrubbed
- 1 large egg
- 80g / scant ⅔ cup gluten-free plain (all-purpose) flour, plus extra for dusting

If you've never made gluten-free pasta before, definitely start with gnocchi. These little fluffy dumplings are super easy to make using just three ingredients. Use them in place of pasta in almost any dish, or in my pepperoni gnocchi bake recipe on page 136.

Preheat your oven to 200°C fan / 220°C / 425°F.

Put your potatoes (unpeeled and whole) on a baking tray and bake in the oven for 45 minutes or until cooked through - poke through the middle with a skewer to check.

Cut each potato in half. As they will be too hot to handle, use a fork to hold them steady and use a spoon to scoop out all of the flesh into a mixing bowl, leaving the skins behind. Don't leave any flesh in the skins - waste not, want not! Mash the flesh until smooth with a fork (hard work) or using a potato masher/ricer (easy and quick). Either way, ensure there are no lumps.

Crack in the egg, gradually add the flour and mix thoroughly. When the mixture begins to come together, use your hands to form a *smooth* ball of dough. It should now have a texture more like dough than mashed potato.

Dough too sticky? Gradually add a little more flour, a teaspoon at a time. Dough too cracked and dry to form a dough ball? Gradually add a teaspoon of water, a few drops at a time.

Place your dough ball onto a *very lightly* floured surface (too much flour will make your cooked gnocchi unpleasantly sticky) and knead for 30 seconds or so.

Divide the dough into two equal portions. Using your hands, roll out one portion into a long sausage shape, about 1.5cm / ½in thick. Cut the dough sausage into 2cm / ¾in sections and roll each piece into a ball. Then, using the back of a fork, lightly rock back and forth over each ball to create a nice ridged pattern (this will help sauce stick to them better). Repeat with the other half of your gnocchi dough.

Bring a large saucepan of water to the boil over a medium heat and add 1 tablespoon of salt. Add a quarter of your gnocchi dumplings to the boiling water and cook for 1 minute or until they all rise to the surface. Remove the gnocchi from the water using a slotted spoon and repeat until all of your gnocchi have been cooked.

TIP:

Using lots of small potatoes isn't ideal for this recipe - they will be much more troublesome to work with when it comes to separating the flesh from the skin!

Shortcrust PASTRY

use a hard dairy-free butter alternative →

(dairy-free) (low fodmap) (low lactose) (vegetarian)

MAKES · ENOUGH TO LINE A 23CM / 9IN PIE DISH

TAKES · 15 MINUTES + 25 MINUTES CHILLING

- 200g / 1½ cups gluten-free plain (all-purpose) flour
- 1 tsp xanthan gum
- 100g / scant ½ cup very cold butter, cut into 1cm / ½in cubes
- 30g / 2½ tbsp caster (superfine) sugar (if making a sweet pastry case)
- 1 large egg, beaten
- 3–5 tsp cold water

This versatile, buttery pastry can be used for either sweet or savoury pies by including or omitting the sugar as needed. Shh... you'd never know it's gluten-free! Use it for my mini chicken, leek and bacon pies (page 130), quiche Lorraine (page 132) or Bakewell tart (page 180).

In a large mixing bowl, mix together your flour and xanthan gum.

Make sure your butter is really cold: if not, put it into the fridge or freezer until nicely chilled, then add to the bowl and mix it into the flour.

Using your fingertips, rub the butter into the flour to form a breadcrumb-like consistency. Make sure your hands are cool as we want to avoid the butter getting warm! Stir in your sugar, if making sweet pastry. Add in your beaten egg and, using a knife, carefully cut it into the mixture. You don't want it to come together just yet, so don't use your hands to push it together, even if it feels like you could.

Add the cold water a teaspoon at a time, using your knife to cut it in. The mixture will start to really come together at this point. I find that, at around 3 teaspoons, it's about the right consistency to push together into a ball with my hands. It should be a little sticky to touch but not unmanageable.

Wrap the dough in cling film (plastic wrap) and leave to chill in the fridge for around 25 minutes before using. You can freeze this pastry for up to 2 months; defrost fully before using.

TIP:
Chill! Using cold water, cold butter and chilling the dough makes your gluten-free pastry stronger and more workable. Making any type of pastry on an incredibly hot day isn't advisable, as the warmer your dough is, the more fragile it will become.

ROUGH PUFF Pastry

MAKES · 650G / 1LB 7OZ

TAKES · 30 MINUTES + 1 HOUR 15 MINUTES CHILLING

- 295g / generous 2 cups gluten-free plain (all-purpose) flour, plus extra for dusting
- 1 tsp xanthan gum
- Pinch of salt
- 225g / 1 cup very cold butter, cut into 1cm / ½in cubes
- 1 egg white
- Ice-cold water

This versatile pastry is light and buttery, with lots of crisp, flaky layers that magically puff up when baked. Use it to make my pastéis de nata, Danish pastries or sausage rolls (pages 182, 183 and 98). This once seemed absolutely impossible to make gluten-free... but here we are!

In a large mixing bowl, mix together your flour, xanthan gum and salt.

Make sure your butter is really cold; if not, put it into the fridge or freezer until nicely chilled. Add your butter to the bowl and stir it into the flour. Gently squeeze the butter with your fingertips, to break the cubes down a little – make sure your hands are cool as we want to avoid the butter getting warm! Definitely don't try and rub them into the flour as we want to see chunks of butter in the mix at all times.

Add your egg white to a jug (pitcher) and add ice-cold water to the jug until the mixture reaches 130ml / 4½fl oz in total. Mix briefly to combine. Gradually add three-quarters of the wet mixture to your mixing bowl, tossing the mixture with your hands, or using a knife to cut it in, between pouring. This will allow the mix to hydrate, but don't try to form a dough at this point.

Once you've added three-quarters of the wet mixture, start to add it in even smaller quantities, still tossing in between. If your dough doesn't start to come together after adding all of it, you might need to add up to an extra 15ml / 1 tablespoon water. Once a dough starts to form, only then begin bringing it together with your hands – you don't want it to be too dry or sticky, just somewhere in between.

Using your hands, form a rectangle with the dough and wrap in cling film (plastic wrap). It should have visible streaks of butter in it. Place in the fridge for about 15 minutes.

Remove your dough from the fridge and remove the cling film. Roll it out on a lightly floured, large piece of non-stick baking parchment until just over 1cm / ½in thick. Fold over the bottom of the dough so it meets the centre, then fold the top of the rolled-out dough over that, like a letter in an envelope. Try your best to get the layers fairly evenly folded, but at this stage, it doesn't matter if it looks messy.

As we need to keep the dough as cold as possible, cover and return to the fridge for about 15 minutes. Repeat the rolling, folding and chilling 3 more times, turning the pastry 90 degrees each time you roll. On its last trip to the fridge, chill it for no less than 30 minutes before using.

You can freeze this pastry for up to 2 months; defrost fully before using.

TIPS:
Chill! Using cold water, cold butter and chilling the dough makes your gluten-free pastry stronger and more workable. Making any type of pastry on an incredibly hot day isn't advisable, as the warmer your dough is, the more fragile it will become.

Remember that when using rough puff pastry, you cannot simply just reroll it (or any offcuts) into a ball. You'll destroy the layers you've spent time creating! If you do have any offcuts, you can always bake them and roll them in cinnamon sugar for a sweet treat.

Making it dairy-free?
Use a (hard) dairy-free alternative to butter. I find that hard margarine is still a little too soft for rough puff, so use a block that feels very firm when chilled.

HOT
WATER
CRUST
Pastry

 use dairy-free milk and lard

 use lactose-free milk

 use lactose-free milk

 use butter instead of lard

**MAKES · ENOUGH FOR
12 MINI PORK PIES**

TAKES · 20 MINUTES

- 500g / 3¾ cups gluten-free plain (all-purpose) flour
- 1 tsp xanthan gum
- 1½ tsp salt
- 2 large eggs
- 170g / ¾ cup lard or butter
- 220ml / 1 cup minus 2 tbsp milk

This pastry is used to make proper British pork pies (try mine on page 97), but you can use it to make any other savoury pie you like. It's characteristically thick, flaky and packed with flavour. Traditionally, hot water crust pastry doesn't contain egg and you'd work with the dough while it's hot, but adding egg and allowing the dough to chill is vital in making this work as a gluten-free equivalent. Fortunately, you'd never even know the difference!

In a large mixing bowl, add your flour, xanthan gum and salt, then make a well in the middle. Beat the eggs in a separate bowl, then add to the well but don't mix them in just yet.

Chop your lard or butter into small chunks and place in a small saucepan over a low-medium heat. As soon as it begins to show signs of melting, add in your milk and slowly heat until all the lard or butter is melted. Stir to ensure everything is well combined.

Add the hot mixture to your mixing bowl and mix immediately until well incorporated. Using your hands, bring together into a ball.

At this point, the dough should be lovely, oily and smooth. Wrap it in cling film (plastic wrap) and pop it into the fridge for 1 hour before using. Chilling adds much needed strength and structure to the dough, so don't skip this part!

You can freeze this pastry for up to 2 months; defrost fully before using.

Choux PASTRY

 use dairy-free milk and a hard dairy-free butter alternative

 use lactose-free milk

 use lactose-free milk

MAKES · ENOUGH FOR 18 PROFITEROLES OR 14 ÉCLAIRS

TAKES · 30 MINUTES

- 150g / 1 cup plus 2 tbsp gluten-free self-raising (self-rising) flour
- ¼ tsp xanthan gum
- 2 tsp caster (superfine) sugar
- ¼ tsp salt
- 150ml / 10 tbsp milk
- 150ml / 10 tbsp water
- 100g / ½ cup minus 1 tbsp butter, cubed
- 4 large eggs, beaten

Choux pastry is one of those rare gems that miraculously works the same from start to finish, with or without gluten. Of course, a little added xanthan gum goes a long way! Use this pastry to pipe profiteroles and chocolate éclairs, then wonder why you didn't make it sooner.

Sift your flour, xanthan gum, sugar and salt into a mixing bowl. Place to one side.

Add your milk, water and cubed butter to a small to medium saucepan and place over a low-medium heat. Gently heat until the butter has melted, then bring to a gentle simmer and, as soon as it is simmering, take off the heat and immediately add your dry mixture to the pan. Mix immediately and vigorously until everything comes together into a dough. If the mixture still seems a tiny bit moist on top, put it back on a very low heat, stirring continuously for a minute or so – don't let it stick to the bottom!

Place the dough in a large mixing bowl and leave to cool for 10 minutes. Once cooled, gradually add your beaten eggs to the dough, mixing thoroughly between each addition until smooth. Watch the consistency of the dough when you add the egg as you don't want it to go too runny – it needs to be thick enough to be a pipeable consistency that can hold its shape, and you might not need all of the egg. You can beat in the egg by hand using a wooden spoon quite easily but it's a proper workout! I use an electric hand whisk on a low speed.

Transfer your dough to a piping bag fitted with an open star nozzle then follow the baking instructions on pages 202 and 204 for my profiteroles or chocolate éclairs.

Ladyfingers
(SAVOIARDI)

MAKES · 12

TAKES · 25 MINUTES

- 3 egg yolks
- 120g / ½ cup plus 1½ tbsp caster (superfine) sugar
- ½ tsp vanilla extract
- 4 egg whites
- 110g / generous ¾ cup gluten-free plain (all-purpose) flour
- 30g / ⅓ cup cornflour (cornstarch)
- ¼ tsp xanthan gum

These sponge fingers are like sweet, fluffy clouds, ready and waiting to soak up tons of flavour. They're perfect for soaking up coffee in my tiramisu (page 201) or sherry in my trifle (page 212). Alternatively, simply dust with icing (confectioners') sugar and dip them in your coffee!

Preheat your oven to 170°C fan / 190°C / 375°F. Line two large baking sheets with non-stick baking parchment.

In a large mixing bowl, add your egg yolks, half of your sugar and the vanilla. Whisk together until combined and lighter in colour.

Whisk the egg whites in a separate bowl until fluffy and white in colour (I use an electric hand whisk or a stand mixer at a medium speed for this). Gradually add the other half of your sugar to the egg whites and keep whisking until it forms stiff peaks. You should be able to put the bowl above your head without anything falling out.

Using a large metal spoon, one large spoonful at a time, very gently fold the stiff egg white into the egg yolk and sugar mixture until it is all combined.

In a separate bowl, mix together the flour, cornflour and xanthan gum, then sift this into your egg mixture. Using a metal spoon, very gently fold in until well combined.

Spoon the mixture into a piping bag (no nozzle needed) and snip off the end. If you don't have a piping bag, you can spoon the mixture into a plastic sandwich bag and snip the corner off. Or carefully spoon the mixture onto your baking sheets in lines as described below. If you only have one large baking sheet, cook the fingers in 2 batches.

Pipe the mixture in lines about 10cm / 4in long onto your prepared baking sheets. Make sure you push the mixture out a little so your lines are not too narrow. Cook in the oven for 15 minutes, then remove from the oven, leave on the trays for 5-10 minutes, then transfer to a wire rack to fully cool.

You can use them on the day you bake them or leave them a few days to harden and go a little stale - weirdly, for once, that's a good thing!

° GLUTEN-FREE °
Breadcrumbs

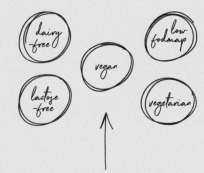

dairy free

lactose free

vegan

low fodmap

vegetarian

ensure the bread is all of these first

MAKES · ABOUT 250G / ABOUT 4 CUPS

TAKES · 10 MINUTES

• 5 slices of white gluten-free bread (page 41 or store-bought)

As I'm sure we all know, gluten-free bread is too expensive to waste! Since stale bread works best here, this is the perfect way to use it up instead of wasting it. Perfect for my katsu curry (page 113) or Scotch eggs (page 96).

Toast all your bread until completely golden and crisp. Lightly toasted bread won't work half as well so make sure they're as golden brown as possible... without burning them, obviously!

Once cooled, grab a large mixing bowl. Either crumble the bread by hand or you can use a food processor to whizz them into nice and even, fine crumbs.

If the breadcrumbs still feel a little soft and bread-like at this point, you can spread them on a baking tray and briefly bake them in a hot oven for 5 minutes until they brown a little more.

Store in an airtight container for up to 1 month.

Lazy Gluten-free GRAVY -

 use a dairy-free butter alternative

 use a low FODMAP stock cube and ensure browning is onion/garlic-free

 use a gluten-free veggie stock cube

MAKES · 400ML / 1⅔ CUPS

TAKES · 10 MINUTES

- 50g / 3½ tbsp butter
- 3 tbsp gluten-free plain (all-purpose) flour
- 500ml / 2 cups gluten-free beef or chicken stock
- ½ tsp gravy browning sauce
- ½ tsp black pepper

It couldn't be easier to make your own gluten-free gravy at home - no meat drippings or gravy granules required. Serve up alongside your Sunday roast dinner and drench those gluten-free Yorkshire puds (page 90)!

Melt your butter in a saucepan over a low-medium heat. Once melted, add your flour and whisk until it forms a smooth paste.

Add in your stock, gravy browning sauce and black pepper and stir in well. Bring to the boil and simmer until it thickens. Allow to cool for 5 minutes as it'll thicken a little more as it cools.

TIP:
You can easily find gravy browning sauce in supermarkets here in the UK and it's gluten-free too. If you can't find it where you live, you can always use a teaspoon of gluten-free dark soy sauce using the recipe on page 35.

Making it vegan?
Use a gluten-free and vegan stock cube, as well as a dairy-free alternative to butter.

Egg Noodles

swap gram flour for more gf flour →

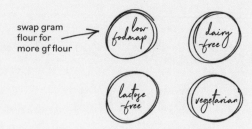

MAKES · 500G / 18OZ COOKED NOODLES (450G / 1LB UNCOOKED)

TAKES · 45 MINUTES

- 230g / 1⅔ cups gluten-free plain (all-purpose) flour, plus extra for dusting
- 50g / ⅖ cup gram (chickpea) flour
- ¼ tsp ground turmeric
- 1 tsp xanthan gum
- 3 large eggs

Gluten-free egg noodles don't exist. Until now! You might notice that this is very similar to my fresh pasta recipe... because it is! Pasta and egg noodles have very similar core ingredients, but the main distinction here is that you need to allow them to air-dry after cooking. Air-drying them gives them that firmer, chewy texture of egg noodles that sets them apart from pasta – use them in my chow mein recipe (page 109).

In a large mixing bowl, add the flour, gram flour, turmeric and xanthan gum. Mix together and make a well in the middle. Add your eggs to the well and mix with a fork until all the egg is incorporated. Use your hands to form a slightly sticky dough ball.

Dough too wet and sloppy? Slowly add 1 teaspoon of extra flour until sticky. Dough too dry to form a ball? Gradually add 1 teaspoon of water. It should be a little sticky at this point.

On a well-floured surface, knead the dough for 1 minute or until it becomes smooth and no longer sticky. Place the dough ball back into the bowl and cover with cling film (plastic wrap). Allow to rest for 30 minutes – don't rush this part as it gives the dough much needed elasticity.

Cut the dough ball into equal quarters and take one portion of the dough. Leave the rest covered in the bowl so they don't dry out. From this point onwards, use as little flour as possible to dust your work surface and rolling pin – only add a little when the dough is sticking.

Using a rolling pin, roll out the dough portion on a *lightly* floured surface to 5mm / ¼in thickness – aim for a long lasagne sheet shape. Fold the rolled-out dough like a book and then fold over once more. The folding is integral as it gives the dough strength and structure.

Roll out the dough for a final time into a long lasagne sheet shape – this time aim for 1mm / 1⁄32in thickness so that it's paper thin and almost see-through. The noodles will double in thickness once cooked, so it's key to get it as thin as possible.

Lightly flour the surface of your rolled-out dough and gently rub it in so that it disappears. Very loosely fold over the bottom of the dough so that it meets the centre. Then loosely fold the top of the rolled-out dough over that. It should be folded up like a letter in an envelope with a little slack on each fold.

Take a long, sharp knife and trim off the untidy edges. Then smoothly cut the folded dough into very thin strips (maximum 2mm / 1⁄16in). Don't 'saw' the dough when cutting as it may tear, and take your time so that they're all a uniform size. Gently unravel your folded strips to reveal long noodles. Place onto your lightly floured surface to avoid them sticking together.

Repeat the rolling and cutting with the rest of your dough.

To cook the noodles

Cook for 4–5 minutes in 2 batches in a large saucepan of boiling water with 1 tablespoon of salt added, then drain. Create 4 nests of noodles and allow to air-dry on a wooden board for 2–3 hours before using – they are now ready to fry, straight to wok. The drying process is key to give the noodles a firm, chewy texture.

To make dried noodles

After cutting your noodles from the rolled-out dough, create 4 nests and allow to dry out for 24 hours on a wooden board, turning them over halfway. You can keep the dried nests in an airtight container in the fridge for up to 5 days. Cook for 5-7 minutes and allow to air-dry on a wooden board for 2-3 hours before using.

TIP:
The less flour you use for dusting, the better. It can make your cooked noodles unpleasantly sticky and starchy. You can also use a pasta machine if you like. Though it isn't necessary, it can help when cutting the noodles.

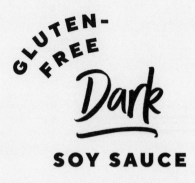

GLUTEN-FREE Dark SOY SAUCE

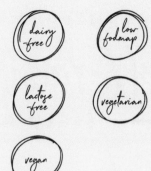

dairy free · low fodmap · lactose free · vegetarian · vegan

MAKES · 400ML / 1²⁄₃ CUPS

TAKES · 15 MINUTES

- 300ml / 1¼ cups gluten-free soy sauce
- 250g / 1¼ cups dark brown sugar
- 2 tbsp cornflour (cornstarch)
- 4 tbsp water

Another essential that literally doesn't exist is gluten-free *dark* soy sauce. And that's even harder to believe when you realize just how simple it is to make. It has a deeper, sweeter taste and, of course, gives your fakeaways that authentic dark soy sauce colour. This is the best use of 15 minutes for anyone who misses all their favourite Chinese takeaway dishes.

Add your soy sauce and sugar to a small saucepan, place over a medium heat and immediately mix so that everything is well combined.

Slowly bring to the boil, stirring occasionally. Once at boiling point, reduce the heat so that it's barely bubbling and allow to simmer for 5 minutes.

Mix together your cornflour and water in a small dish. Drizzle it into the soy mixture in the pan, whisking constantly to avoid lumps. Continue to simmer for another 5–10 minutes, then remove from the heat. Allow the mixture to reach room temperature. It will thicken slightly more as it cools.

Store in a bottle or jar in the fridge for up to 2 months.

GLUTEN-FREE
Self-raising flour
(SELF-RISING)

MAKES · 450G / 3¼ CUPS

TAKES · 2 MINUTES

- 450g / 3¼ cups gluten-free plain (all-purpose) flour
- 6 tsp gluten-free baking powder
- 1 tsp xanthan gum

Gluten-free self-raising flour is available across all supermarkets in the UK, but if you can't find it where you live, you can easily make your own using the ratios here. Can't find gluten-free plain flour? Head over to my blog to find out how to create your own blend.

Simply combine all the ingredients in a mixing bowl and mix thoroughly. It might be wise to double the quantities to ensure you don't have to make it too often.

Store in a large airtight container. Consider labelling it so you can tell it apart from other flour!

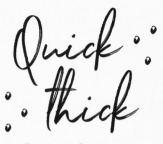

Quick thick
CUSTARD

use dairy-free milk instead of the milk and cream

use lactose-free milk instead of the milk and cream

use lactose-free milk instead of the milk and cream

MAKES · 500ML / 2 CUPS

TAKES · 10 MINUTES

- 250ml / 1 cup whole milk
- 250ml / 1 cup double (heavy) cream
- 5 egg yolks
- 40g / scant ¼ cup caster (superfine) sugar
- 2 tsp cornflour (cornstarch)
- 2 tsp vanilla extract

You simply cannot beat fresh, thick custard served up alongside all your favourite desserts. My method comes very close to beating custard powder in terms of convenience too – so there's no need to stir for ages until your arm falls off!

Add your milk and cream to a large saucepan and place over a medium heat.

In a medium mixing bowl, whisk together your egg yolks, sugar, cornflour and vanilla extract until well combined.

Once the milk and cream mixture has reached just before boiling point, gradually pour it into your egg and sugar mixture, whisking constantly until well combined.

Return the mixture to the (cleaned) saucepan over a medium heat and bring to the boil, whisking constantly. Simmer and it should thicken immediately, but if not, keep whisking until it does. Once thickened, serve with your favourite desserts.

TIPS:

If you wish to keep your custard for later, or you're using it to make the trifle on page 212, pour into a glass bowl or jug (pitcher) and cover the surface with cling film (plastic wrap) so that it touches the custard, and allow to cool. Store in the fridge for up to 2 days before using.

If you like your custard to be even sweeter you can add a little more sugar than I suggest.

Making it vegan?
Use dairy-free milk in place of the milk and cream and leave out the egg yolks. Combine everything in a saucepan and add 4 tbsp cornflour instead of 2 tsp. Place over a low heat and don't stop stirring until it thickens. Add a tiny pinch of ground turmeric to achieve a nice custard colour, if you like.

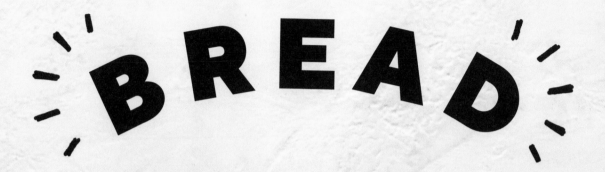

BREAD

All I wanted was gluten-free bread that actually tasted like 'real' fresh bread, and after years of perfecting, I finally did it – I didn't believe it was even possible myself, to be quite honest!

So here's everything from a crusty white sandwich loaf, to artisan boules, French baguettes, Peshwari naan bread and more. I promise that you'd never know they were gluten-free and you'll probably save yourself a lot of money by baking them yourself. As with most bread, the loaves on these pages are best enjoyed fresh on the day they are baked, but will last 2–3 days stored in an airtight container. Most are also perfect for slicing and freezing.

This is the only chapter of this book where a small handful of recipes may require one or two very specific additions (like psyllium husk powder, see page 14) that you can't ordinarily find in the supermarket. If you really miss bread as much as I did, I'm sure you'll have no hesitation in hopping online and ordering them! Trust me – you'll be glad that you did.

So get ready to be reminded of what 'real' bread tastes like.

PS: I can't emphasize how important it is to weigh out your ingredients with digital cooking scales when baking gluten-free bread. The difference of 10 grams or millilitres can make a huge difference!

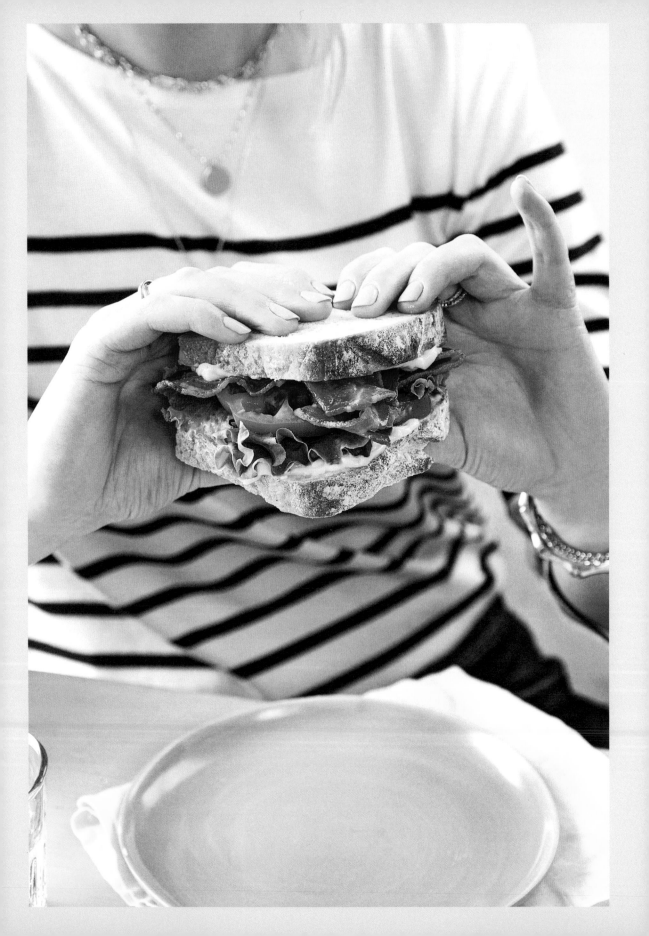

Crusty White
SANDWICH LOAF

low fodmap

lactose free

vegetarian

dairy free

use oil for greasing

**MAKES · 1 LOAF
(ABOUT 15 SLICES)**

**TAKES · 1 HOUR
10 MINUTES + 30-45
MINUTES PROVING**

- 475ml / scant 2 cups warm water
- 10g / ⅓oz active dried yeast (ensure gluten-free)
- 25g / 2 tbsp caster (superfine) sugar
- 180g / scant 1½ cups gluten-free rice flour
- 190g / scant 1½ cups gluten-free plain (all-purpose) flour, plus extra for dusting
- 2 tsp xanthan gum
- 25g / 1oz psyllium husk powder (ensure gluten-free)
- 6g / ¼oz salt
- 2 tsp cider vinegar
- 80g / 3oz egg white (about 2 large eggs)
- Butter or oil, for greasing

For years, I believed that gluten-free bread always had to taste worse than 'real' bread. But after trying bread at some of the game-changing gluten-free bakeries in Barcelona, I realized that anything was possible! With a wonderful crusty exterior and an exceptionally soft and springy middle, I finally made a loaf that I can honestly say doesn't taste gluten-free at all.

In a jug (pitcher), stir together your warm water, yeast and sugar. Allow to stand for 10 minutes until nice and frothy.

In a large bowl or the bowl of a stand mixer, add both flours, the xanthan gum, psyllium husk powder and salt. Mix together until well combined, then add your vinegar, egg white and frothy yeast mixture to the dry ingredients.

Either in a stand mixer fitted with a beater attachment or using an electric hand whisk, mix on a high speed for 3-5 minutes until well combined. It should look like a very thick, sticky batter. Allow to rest for about 10 minutes - this bread batter is very wet, and resting it is super important.

Lightly grease a bread tin (pan), about 26 x 12cm / 10 x 4¾in, and line with non-stick baking parchment.

Pour your rested mixture into the lined tin, ensuring that it's nicely smoothed out and level. Loosely cover with cling film (plastic wrap) and leave to prove in a warm place for 30-45 minutes, until noticeably risen. Proving can take longer on a cold day, so keep an eye on your loaf!

Preheat your oven to 240°C fan / 260°C / 500°F (or as hot as your oven will go if it doesn't reach these temperatures). Place a large roasting dish at the bottom of the oven and boil a kettle.

Dust the top of your loaf with a little flour and slash the top of the dough three times using a sharp knife. Place in the preheated oven and immediately add a mug's worth of boiling water to the roasting dish. Bake for 20 minutes, then reduce the oven temperature to 200°C fan / 220°C / 425°F and bake for another 30 minutes, until golden brown.

Remove from the oven. Carefully remove from the tin and tap the base to check that it feels and sounds hollow - if so, then it's done. Place onto a wire rack and allow to cool completely before slicing.

TIP:
If you want an even crustier crust, once the loaf is cooked, remove it from the tin and allow it to cool in the warm (switched off) oven with the door open.

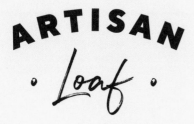

ARTISAN Loaf

**MAKES · 1 LOAF
(ABOUT 15 SLICES)**

**TAKES · 1 HOUR
10 MINUTES + 30–45
MINUTES PROVING**

- 475ml / scant 2 cups warm water
- 10g / ⅓oz active dried yeast (ensure gluten-free)
- 25g / 2 tbsp caster (superfine) sugar
- 180g / 1½ cups gluten-free buckwheat flour
- 190g / scant 1½ cups gluten-free plain (all-purpose) flour, plus extra for dusting
- 2 tsp xanthan gum
- 25g / 1oz psyllium husk powder (ensure gluten-free)
- 6g / ¼oz salt
- 2 tsp cider vinegar
- 80g / 3oz egg white (about 2 large eggs)
- Pumpkin seeds and poppy seeds, to sprinkle (optional)

I never thought I'd be able to eat a loaf that looked and tasted like this, let alone bake one myself! It's lovely and crusty, but with that unmistakable light and airy crumb, packed with tons of wholegrain flavour thanks to the seeds and buckwheat.

In a jug (pitcher), stir together your warm water, yeast and sugar. Allow to stand for 10 minutes until nice and frothy.

In a large bowl or the bowl of a stand mixer, add both flours, the xanthan gum, psyllium husk powder and salt. Mix together until well combined, then add your vinegar, egg white and frothy yeast mixture to the dry ingredients.

Either in a stand mixer fitted with a beater attachment or using an electric hand whisk, mix on a high speed for 3–5 minutes until well combined. It should look like a very thick, sticky batter. Allow to rest for about 10 minutes – this bread batter is very wet, and resting it is super important.

Grab a proving basket and add 1 tablespoon of flour to it. Rotate the basket so that the flour lightly coats all of the base and sides. Pour your mixture into the prepared basket, ensuring that it's nicely smoothed out and level. Loosely cover with cling film (plastic wrap) and allow to prove in a warm place for 30–45 minutes until noticeably risen.

Proving can take longer on a cold day, so keep an eye on your loaf!

Preheat your oven to 240°C fan / 260°C / 500°F (or as hot as your oven will go if it doesn't reach these temperatures). Place a large roasting dish at the bottom of the oven and boil a kettle.

Once your dough has risen, carefully invert the dough out onto a large sheet of non-stick baking parchment in one quick motion. Use the parchment to gently transfer the dough into a 28cm / 11in skillet or round baking tin (pan).

If using seeds, brush the top of the dough with a little water and sprinkle your seeds on top. If you're omitting the seeds, dust the top of your loaf with a little flour. Slash the top of the dough three times using a sharp knife, transfer to the preheated oven and immediately add a mug's worth of boiling water to the roasting dish. Bake for 20 minutes, then reduce the oven temperature to 200°C fan / 220°C / 425°F and bake for another 30 minutes, until a darker brown.

Remove from the oven. Carefully remove from the skillet or tin and tap the base to check that it feels and sounds hollow – if so, then it's done. Place onto a wire rack and allow to cool completely before slicing.

TIP:
You could also bake this in a loaf tin (pan) – see the 'useful equipment' section on page 18 for the correct size tin that you'll need.

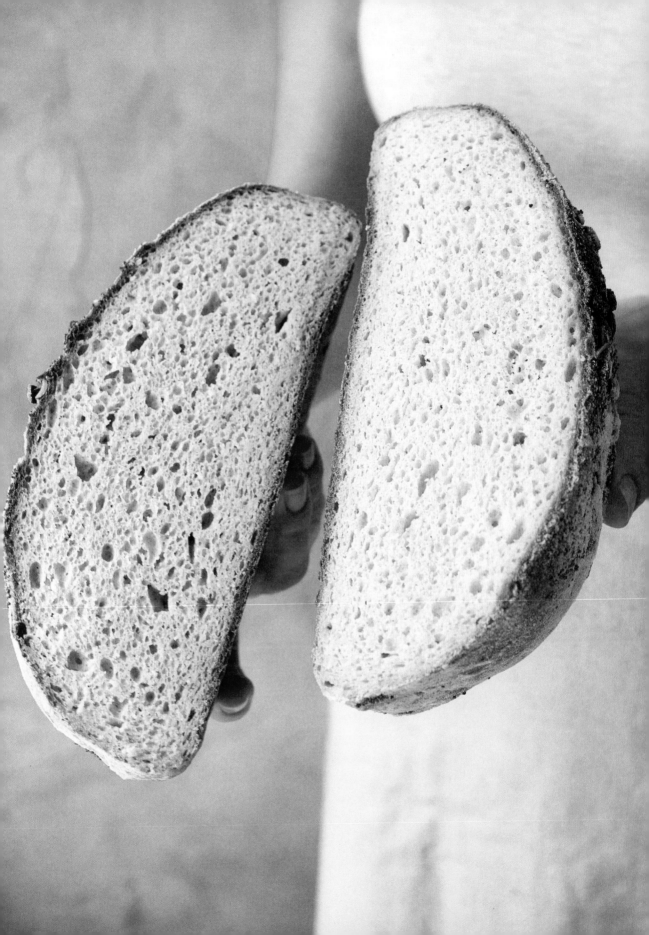

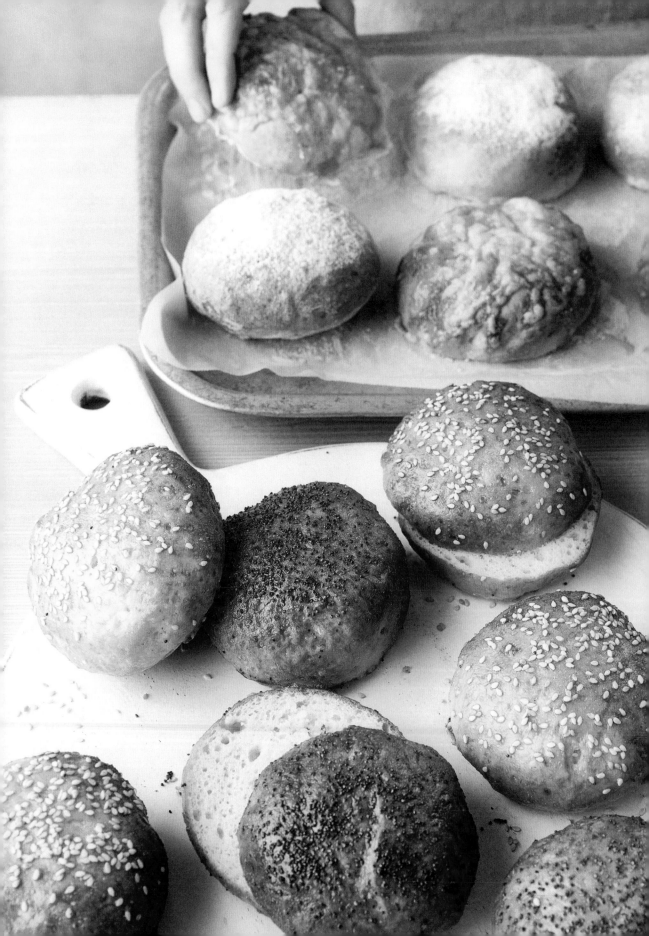

Cheesy or Floured BAPS

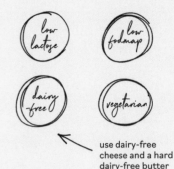

use dairy-free cheese and a hard dairy-free butter alternative

MAKES · 6-8

TAKES · 1 HOUR + 45-60 MINUTES PROVING

- 330ml / 1⅜ cups warm water
- 10g / ⅓oz active dried yeast (ensure gluten-free)
- 25g / 2 tbsp caster (superfine) sugar
- 410g / 3 cups gluten-free white bread flour or gluten-free plain (all-purpose) flour, plus extra for dusting
- 2 tsp xanthan gum
- 15g / ½oz psyllium husk powder (ensure gluten-free)
- 6g / ¼oz salt
- 1 tsp cider vinegar
- 3 egg whites
- 30g / 2 tbsp butter, melted
- 50g / 1¾oz extra mature Cheddar cheese, grated (optional)

These bread rolls are wonderfully soft and light with a crusty finish. I never get tired of squeezing them and watching them spring right back into shape! Finish with cheese or a dusting of flour - the choice is yours!

Line a baking tray with non-stick baking parchment.

In a jug (pitcher), stir together your warm water, yeast and sugar. Allow to stand for 10 minutes until nice and frothy.

In a large bowl or the bowl of a stand mixer, add your flour, xanthan gum, psyllium husk powder and salt. Mix together until well combined, then add your vinegar, egg whites, melted butter and frothy yeast mixture to the dry ingredients.

Either in a stand mixer fitted with a beater attachment or using an electric hand whisk, mix on a high speed for 3-5 minutes until well combined. It should look like a very thick, sticky batter. Allow to rest for about 10 minutes - this bread batter is very wet, and resting it is super important.

Flour your work surface and your hands, then divide the rested dough into 6-8 portions that are 140g / 5oz each - I pull off portions straight from the bowl one at a time and place cling film (plastic wrap) on the scales to avoid them sticking.

Transfer one portion of the sticky dough to the floured surface and roll it lightly in the flour so that it's no longer sticky. Mould it with your hands into a round, flat shape then place on your prepared baking tray. Repeat with the rest of your pieces of dough, spacing them apart. Loosely cover with cling film and allow to prove in a warm place for 45-60 minutes until doubled in size.

Preheat your oven to 200°C fan / 220°C / 425°F. Place a large roasting dish at the bottom of the oven and boil a kettle.

Remove the cling film, brush the proved buns with a little water, then sprinkle over the grated cheese or, alternatively, a dusting of flour. Place the tray in the preheated oven and immediately add a mug's worth of boiling water to the roasting dish. Bake for 20-22 minutes until golden brown, then remove from the oven and allow to cool briefly on the tray before transferring to a wire rack to cool completely.

If not eaten on the same day as baking, these can be refreshed in the microwave or oven.

BRIOCHE-STYLE
Burger Buns

 use dairy-free milk and a hard dairy-free butter alternative

 use lactose-free milk

 use lactose-free milk

MAKES · 8

TAKES · 1 HOUR + 45–60 MINUTES PROVING

- 250ml / 1 cup milk, warmed
- 100ml / generous ⅓ cup water, warmed
- 10g / ⅓oz active dried yeast (ensure gluten-free)
- 25g / 2 tbsp caster (superfine) sugar
- 410g / 3 cups gluten-free white bread flour or gluten-free plain (all-purpose) flour, plus extra for dusting
- 2 tsp xanthan gum
- 15g / ½oz psyllium husk powder (ensure gluten-free)
- 6g / ¼oz salt
- 2 large eggs
- 1 tsp cider vinegar
- 30g / 2 tbsp butter, melted

To finish
- 1 egg, beaten
- Sesame seeds or poppy seeds
- 25g / 1¾ tbsp butter, melted

Over the years I've eaten burgers with either a) buns that fall apart as you eat them or, even worse, b) no bun at all. But when these burger buns are like a fluffy cloud in the middle with that unmistakable glossy exterior, there's no excuse to miss out on enjoying a delicious burger like everybody else!

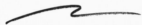

Line a baking tray with non-stick baking parchment.

Mix your warm milk and water, yeast and sugar in a jug (pitcher). Allow to stand for 10 minutes until nice and frothy.

In a large bowl or the bowl of a stand mixer, add your flour, xanthan gum, psyllium husk powder and salt. Mix together until well combined then add your eggs, vinegar, melted butter and frothy yeast mixture to the dry ingredients.

Either in a stand mixer fitted with a beater attachment or with an electric hand whisk, mix on a high speed for 3–5 minutes until well combined. It should look like a very thick, sticky batter. Allow to rest for about 10 minutes.

Flour your work surface and your hands and divide the dough into 8 portions, each about 110g / scant 4oz – I pull off portions straight from the bowl one at a time and place cling film (plastic wrap) on the scales so they don't stick. Transfer each portion to the floured surface and roll lightly in the flour so that it's no longer sticky. Mould it with your hands into a round, flat shape then place on your prepared baking tray, spacing them apart.

Loosely cover with cling film and allow to prove in a warm place for 45–60 minutes until doubled in size.

Preheat your oven to 200°C fan / 220°C / 425°F. Place a large roasting dish at the bottom of the oven and boil the kettle.

Remove the cling film, brush the buns with beaten egg and sprinkle with sesame or poppy seeds, then transfer the tray to the preheated oven and immediately add a mug's worth of boiling water to the roasting dish. Bake for 20–22 minutes until golden brown, then remove from the oven and immediately brush with melted butter. Transfer to a wire rack to cool completely.

If not eaten on the same day as baking, these can be refreshed in the microwave or oven.

Pictured on page 44

3-Ingredient PIZZA DOUGH

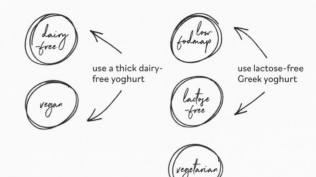

dairy free
vegan
→ use a thick dairy-free yoghurt

low fodmap
lactose-free
→ use lactose-free Greek yoghurt

vegetarian

MAKES · 500G / 18OZ DOUGH

TAKES · 15 MINUTES + 30 MINUTES RESTING

- 250g / generous 1¾ cups gluten-free self-raising (self-rising) flour, plus extra for dusting
- 260g / 1¼ cups Greek yoghurt (or any thick, plain yoghurt)
- ¼ tsp xanthan gum
- Pinch of salt

Did you know that using three simple ingredients, you can throw together pizza dough that nobody would ever know is gluten-free? It also doesn't need any yeast or proving, so it only takes 15 minutes to make. Though it contains yoghurt, people are always surprised to find that it has zero yoghurt taste at all – it simply tastes like 'real' pizza dough!

In a large mixing bowl, add your flour, yoghurt (give it a good stir before using), xanthan gum and salt. Mix together using a spatula and, as it starts to come together, use your hands to bring it together into a slightly sticky ball.

On a well-floured surface, knead the dough briefly until smooth, combined and no longer sticky. Dough still too sticky? Add a little more flour. Dough too dry? Add a little more yoghurt. Cover the dough and allow to rest for 30 minutes.

Use for my gluten-free pizza (page 118) or for my gluten-free calzone (page 139). The unrolled dough can also be chilled and stored in an airtight container to use the next day. Or you can freeze it.

TIPS:
If using a different type of yoghurt that isn't quite as thick, simply add a little more flour to compensate.

You can use this dough to make doughballs, but they work better with yeast – check out the recipe for my cheesy doughballs on page 87.

Pictured on page 119

6-INGREDIENT
Soda Bread

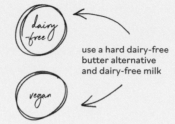

use a hard dairy-free butter alternative and dairy-free milk

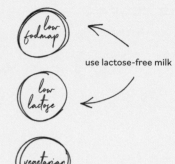

use lactose-free milk

**MAKES · 1 LOAF
(ABOUT 12 SLICES)**

**TAKES · 1 HOUR
30 MINUTES**

- 345ml / 1½ cups minus 1 tbsp milk
- 5 tbsp lemon juice
- 300g / 2¼ cups gluten-free plain (all-purpose) flour, plus extra for dusting
- 1 tsp xanthan gum
- 1 tsp bicarbonate of soda (baking soda)
- ½ tsp salt (optional)
- 30g / 2 tbsp cold butter, cubed

Who knew that you could turn six humble ingredients into freshly baked gluten-free soda bread? There's no yeast required for this recipe, so it's pretty quick as far as bread making goes. It has a soft crust and a lovely, light texture in the middle. If you're new to baking gluten-free bread, this is a great place to start.

Add your milk and lemon juice to a jug (pitcher) and briefly mix. Allow to stand for 10–15 minutes until the mixture becomes thicker and a little lumpy.

In a large mixing bowl, add your flour, xanthan gum, bicarb, and salt, if using, and mix until well combined. Add your butter and rub it in with your fingers until it forms a breadcrumb-like consistency. Pour in your thickened milk mixture and stir well with a wooden spoon, until smooth and it resembles a thick cake batter.

If using a proving basket, add 1 tablespoon of flour to it. Rotate the basket so that the flour lightly coats all of the base and sides. If you don't have a proving basket, prepare a small mixing bowl by greasing the insides with butter. Then add 1 tablespoon of flour to it and rotate the bowl so that the flour lightly coats all of the base and halfway up the sides too.

Pour your mixture into the prepared proving basket or bowl and smooth over the top so it's nice and flat. Cover and allow to rest for no less than 30 minutes.

Preheat the oven to 240°C fan / 260°C / 500°F (or as hot as your oven will go if it doesn't reach these temperatures) and place a 28cm / 11in skillet or round baking tin (pan) in the oven. Place a large roasting dish at the bottom of the oven and boil a kettle.

Once your dough has rested, carefully invert it out onto a large sheet of non-stick baking parchment in one quick motion.

Remove the skillet or baking tin from the oven. Use the baking parchment to gently transfer the dough into the hot skillet or tin. Score a cross in the top of your dough using a sharp knife.

Place in the preheated oven and immediately add a mug's worth of boiling water to the roasting dish. Bake for 10 minutes, then reduce the oven temperature to 200°C fan / 220°C / 425°F and bake for another 30 minutes, until golden. Remove from the oven and carefully remove the loaf from the skillet or baking tin; tap the base to check that it feels and sounds hollow – if so, then it's done. Dust off any excess flour from the top, place onto a wire rack and allow to cool completely before slicing.

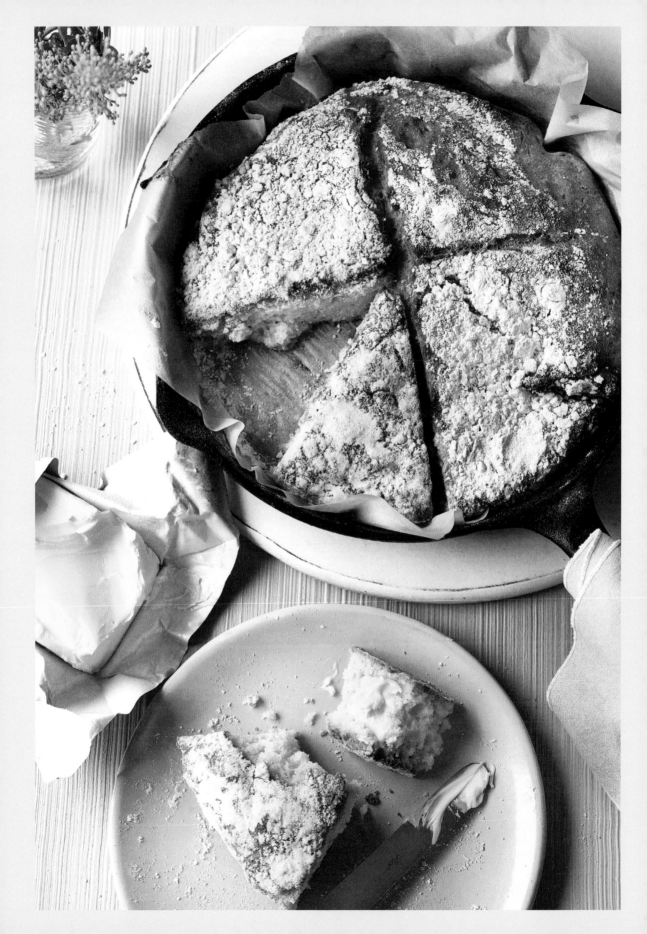

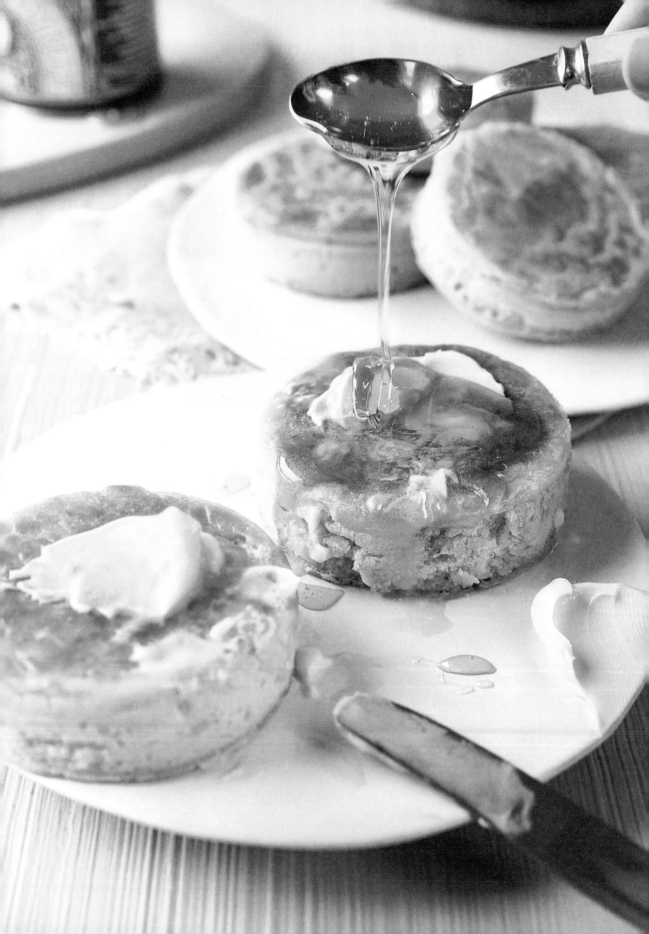

5-INGREDIENT
Crumpets

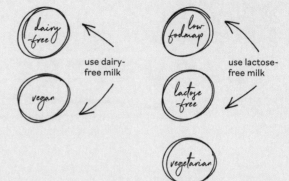

use dairy-free milk

use lactose-free milk

MAKES · 10

TAKES · 30 MINUTES + 1 HOUR PROVING

- 400ml / 1⅔ cups milk, warmed
- 2 tsp caster (superfine) sugar
- 1 tbsp active dried yeast (ensure gluten-free)
- 300g / 2¼ cups gluten-free self-raising (self-rising) flour
- ½ tsp bicarbonate of soda (baking soda)
- ½ tsp salt
- Vegetable oil, for cooking

Does it get any more British than tea and crumpets? Not only would you never know that these are gluten-free, but you wouldn't believe how good freshly baked, homemade crumpets taste.

Stir your warm milk, sugar and yeast together in a jug (pitcher), then allow to stand for 10 minutes until nice and frothy.

In a large mixing bowl, add your flour, bicarb and salt. Add the frothy yeasted milk mixture and mix for 2 minutes until smooth (I use an electric hand whisk for this).

Cover and leave to prove in a warm place for no less than an hour, ideally for 1 hour 30 minutes. There should be some air bubbles on top.

Your mixture should have thickened to an almost pourable consistency. If it has thickened too much, simply add 1–2 tablespoons of warm water to your bowl and mix in.

Add a little vegetable oil to a large frying pan and place over a medium heat. Place either round egg rings or round metal biscuit (cookie) cutters to the pan (you will need to cook the crumpets in batches, depending on how many rings you can fit in the pan).

Spoon 2½ tablespoons of the batter into each ring and cook for about 5 minutes, until little air bubbles appear on the surface and the surface is no longer wet. Using tongs, remove the rings and then flip the crumpets onto the other side to cook for about a minute. Remove from the pan and repeat until you've used up all of your batter.

Serve with butter or a dairy-free alternative, golden syrup, jam (jelly), or whatever takes your fancy.

French
BAGUETTES

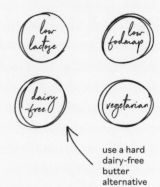

use a hard
dairy-free
butter
alternative

MAKES · 2

TAKES · 1 HOUR + 45 MINUTES PROVING

- 330ml / 1⅜ cups warm water
- 10g / ⅓oz active dried yeast (ensure gluten-free)
- 25g / 2 tbsp caster (superfine) sugar
- 410g / 3 cups gluten-free white bread flour or gluten-free plain (all-purpose) flour
- 2 tsp xanthan gum
- 15g / ½oz psyllium husk powder (ensure gluten-free)
- 6g / ¼oz salt
- 1 tsp cider vinegar
- 3 egg whites
- 30g / 2 tbsp butter, melted, plus extra for greasing
- Sesame seeds or poppy seeds, to sprinkle

Sharing how to make gluten-free baguettes in my very own recipe book was firmly below 'when pigs fly' in my list of things that might one day happen. But here we are! With a golden crust and a soft, white and fluffy middle, I'm still in disbelief that they genuinely taste like the real deal. You'll need a baguette tray to make these, but if you're like me, you'll let nothing stand in the way of you and a French baguette.

In a jug (pitcher), stir together your warm water, yeast and sugar. Allow to stand for 10 minutes until nice and frothy.

In a large bowl or the bowl of a stand mixer, add your flour, xanthan gum, psyllium husk powder and salt. Mix together until well combined, then add your vinegar, egg whites, melted butter and frothy yeast mixture to the dry ingredients.

Either in a stand mixer fitted with a beater attachment or using an electric hand whisk, mix on a high speed for 3–5 minutes until well combined; it should look like a very thick, sticky batter. Allow to rest for about 10 minutes.

Prepare your baguette tray by greasing it with a little butter and sprinkling the base with either sesame or poppy seeds.

Evenly divide your mixture between the two recesses on the baguette tray. As the mixture is fairly sticky, I'd recommend first wetting your fingers and a palette knife, then using them to smooth and shape the batter until you achieve two long baguette shapes. Loosely cover with cling film (plastic wrap) and allow to prove in a warm place for 45 minutes until noticeably risen.

Preheat your oven to 200°C fan / 220°C / 425°F. Place a large roasting dish at the bottom of the oven and boil a kettle.

Once your baguettes are risen, remove the cling film and sprinkle with some additional sesame or poppy seeds. Slash the baguettes 3 or 4 times diagonally using a sharp knife, place in the preheated oven and immediately add a mug's worth of boiling water to the roasting dish. Bake for 20 minutes, then reduce the oven temperature to 160°C fan / 180°C / 350°F and bake for another 20 minutes, until golden brown. If your baguettes are browning a little too much, cover with some foil (shiny side up) for the last 10 minutes.

Remove from the oven and allow to cool briefly in the baguette tray before transferring to a wire rack to cool completely.

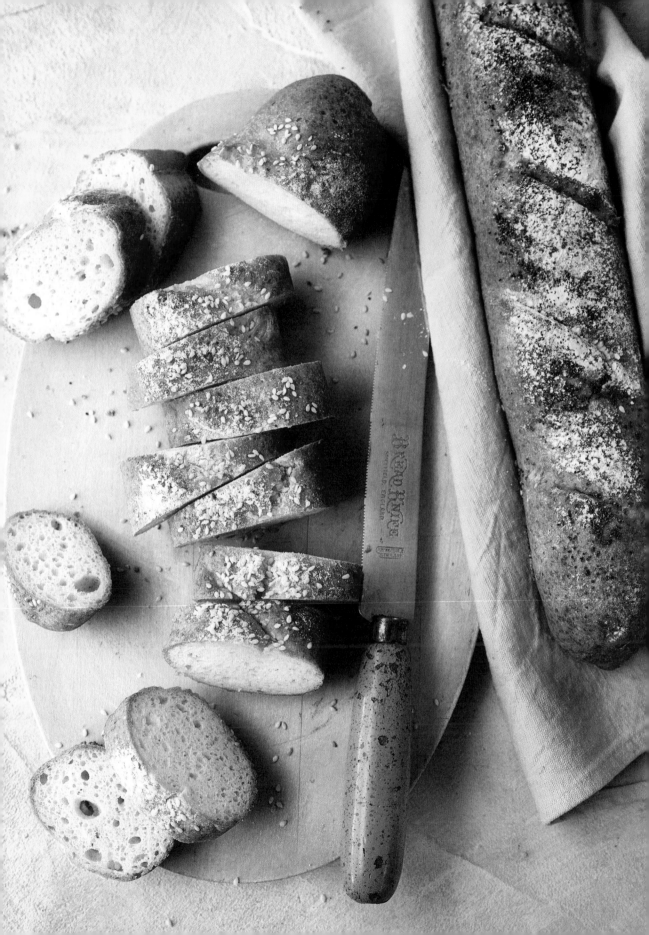

GARLIC AND ROSEMARY
Focaccia

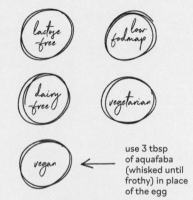

use 3 tbsp
of aquafaba
(whisked until
frothy) in place
of the egg

SERVES · 4–5

**TAKES · 45 MINUTES
+ 1 HOUR PROVING**

- 280ml / 1 cup plus 2 tbsp warm water
- 7g / ¼oz active dried yeast (ensure gluten-free)
- 15g / 1 tbsp caster (superfine) sugar
- 260g / 2 cups gluten-free white bread flour or gluten-free plain (all-purpose) flour
- 2 tsp xanthan gum
- 15g / ½oz psyllium husk powder (ensure gluten-free)
- 6g / ¼oz salt
- 1 large egg
- 1 tsp cider vinegar
- 60ml / ¼ cup olive oil, plus extra for greasing

To finish
- Garlic-infused oil
- Fresh rosemary sprigs
- Maldon (flaky) sea salt

Every time I take a bite of this focaccia, I absolutely cannot believe that it's gluten-free, despite having made it myself! It's light and fluffy in the middle with a soft crust, infused with tons of flavour thanks to the olive oil and finished with a hit of fresh rosemary and salt.

Mix your warm water, yeast and sugar in a jug (pitcher), then allow to stand for 10 minutes until nice and frothy.

In a large bowl or the bowl of a stand mixer, add your flour, xanthan gum, psyllium husk powder and salt. Mix together until well combined, then add your egg, vinegar, oil and frothy yeast mixture to the dry ingredients.

Either in a stand mixer fitted with a beater attachment or with an electric hand whisk, mix on a high speed for 3 minutes until well combined. It should look like a very thick, sticky batter. Leave to rest for about 10 minutes.

Grease a 23cm / 9in square baking tin (pan) with a little oil, then add another glug of olive oil to lightly coat the base of the tin.

Tip your rested dough into the tin and spread out using lightly oiled hands and a spatula. It might seem a little resistant at first, but continue to spread it into a nice, even layer. Loosely cover with cling film (plastic wrap) and prove in a warm place for 1 hour until noticeably risen.

Preheat your oven to 210°C fan / 230°C / 450°F.

Using oiled fingers, make several deep dimples in the risen dough, then drizzle garlic-infused oil all over the top to fill the dimples. Sprinkle with fresh rosemary and salt before cooking in the oven for 25–30 minutes until golden in colour.

Remove from the oven and carefully remove from the baking tin. Tap the base to check that it feels and sounds hollow – if so, then it's done. Drizzle with some extra garlic-infused oil and place onto a wire rack to cool completely before slicing.

TIP:
Feel free to add any extras to the top of your focaccia just before baking – olives and cherry tomatoes work especially well!

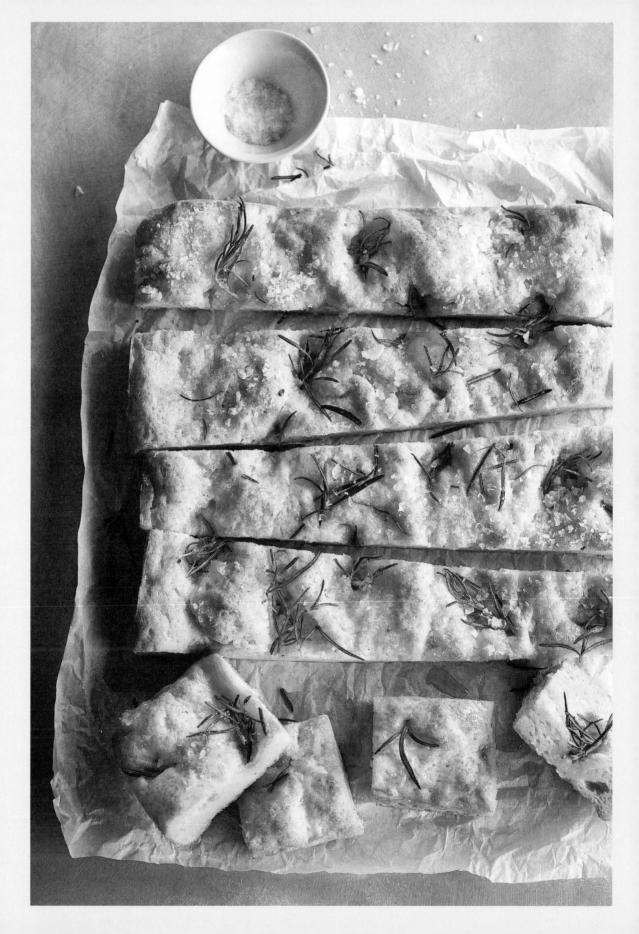

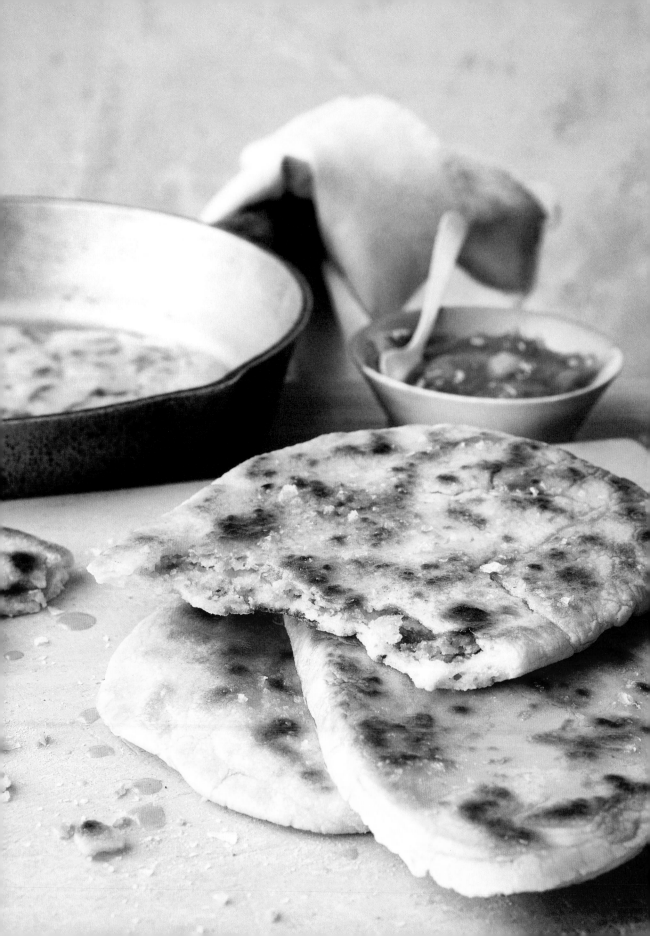

Peshwari
NAAN BREAD

use a thick dairy-free yoghurt and a dairy-free alternative to butter

use lactose-free Greek yoghurt and 28g (1oz) sultanas

use lactose-free Greek yoghurt

MAKES · 4

**TAKES · 20 MINUTES
+ 30 MINUTES RESTING**

- 250g / generous 1¾ cups gluten-free self-raising (self-rising) flour, plus extra for dusting
- 260g / 1¼ cups Greek yoghurt (or any thick, plain yoghurt)
- 1 tsp gluten-free baking powder
- Garlic-infused oil, to serve
- Pinch of salt

For the filling

- 50g / ½ cup ground almonds
- 40g / ⅓ cup sultanas (golden raisins)
- 2 tbsp desiccated (dried shredded) coconut
- 1 tbsp sugar
- 30g / 2 tbsp butter, melted
- 1 tbsp water

Beautifully soft, flexible gluten-free naans are only ever a few simple ingredients away. Filled with a sweet and coconutty filling, these are the ultimate sidekick to any creamy curry. You can also make these without the filling for plain naans, or sprinkle with chopped coriander (cilantro) for garlic and coriander naans.

In a large mixing bowl, add your flour, yoghurt (give it a good stir before using) and baking powder. Mix using a spatula and, as it starts to come together, use your hands to bring it into a slightly sticky ball. Dough still too sticky? Add a little more flour. Dough too dry? Add a little more yoghurt.

On a well-floured surface, knead the dough briefly until smooth, combined and no longer sticky. Cover the dough and allow it to rest for 30 minutes.

For the filling, add all the filling ingredients to a food processor and blitz until it creates a finely blended paste.

Once your dough has rested, place it on a lightly floured surface and divide into 4 equal portions. Use a rolling pin to roll out one dough portion to a 5mm/ ¼in thickness, aiming for an oval shape.

Spread a thin layer of the filling paste on one side of your rolled-out dough, taking care not to tear it, then fold the dough over like a book. Roll out once again into a teardrop shape, 5mm / ¼in thick. If the edges are a little cracked, use your fingers to gently shape them until smooth.

Place a large frying pan over a high heat. The higher the heat, the more bubbles you'll get in the naan. Carefully transfer your naan to the dry pan, using a cake lifter or pizza peel. Cook on one side for 2 minutes or until nicely browned, then flip and cook for 1 minute on the other side, pressing down firmly on the naan using a spatula (this encourages it to puff up a little). Repeat with the remaining dough portions and filling.

Brush with garlic-infused oil, sprinkle on a little salt and serve alongside your favourite curries.

TIPS:
These are freezer-friendly! Simply freeze once cooled and bake in the oven from frozen for 5–8 minutes.

You can make these naan breads plain by removing the filling and/or flavouring them however you like.

2-INGREDIENT
Flatbreads

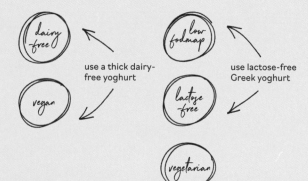

use a thick dairy-free yoghurt

use lactose-free Greek yoghurt

MAKES · 4

**TAKES · 15 MINUTES
+ 30 MINUTES RESTING**

- 250g / generous 1¾ cups gluten-free self-raising (self-rising) flour, plus extra for dusting
- 260g / 1¼ cups Greek yoghurt (or any thick, plain yoghurt)
- Pinch of salt

Did you know that you can make flatbreads that nobody would ever know were gluten-free, from just 2 simple ingredients? This is probably the cheapest and easiest way to make gluten-free bread and, not surprisingly, my freezer is full of them.

In a large mixing bowl, add your flour, yoghurt (give it a good stir before using) and a pinch of salt. Mix using a spatula and, as it starts to come together, use your hands to bring it into a slightly sticky ball. Dough still too sticky? Add a little more flour. Dough too dry? Add a little more yoghurt.

On a well-floured surface, knead the dough briefly until smooth, combined and no longer sticky. Place back into the bowl, cover and allow to rest for 30 minutes.

Transfer your rested dough to a lightly floured surface and divide into 4 equal portions. Use a rolling pin to roll out one dough portion to a 3mm / ⅛in thickness, aiming for an oval shape. If the edges are a little cracked, use your fingers to gently shape the edges until smooth.

Place a large frying pan over a high heat. Once heated, carefully transfer your flatbread into the dry pan, using a cake lifter or pizza peel. Cook on one side for 2 minutes or until nicely browned, then flip and cook for 1 minute on the other side, pressing down firmly using a spatula (this encourages the flatbread to puff up a little). Repeat using the remaining dough portions.

Serve up with my one-pot campfire stew (page 129) and DIY doner kebab (page 124).

TIP:
These are freezer-friendly! Simply freeze once cooled and bake in the oven from frozen for 5–8 minutes.

2-Ingredient CORN TORTILLA WRAPS

MAKES · 12

TAKES · 25 MINUTES

- 200g / 1⅔ cups masa harina flour (blue, yellow or white)
- Pinch of salt
- 350ml / 1½ cups warm water

Did you know that traditional Mexican corn tortillas are naturally gluten-free? All you need is masa harina – a special type of cornflour that you can easily buy online. You'd never know they're gluten-free... because they're always gluten-free! Having a tortilla press helps speed up the process, but certainly isn't mandatory.

In a large mixing bowl, combine the masa harina flour and salt. Add the warm water, mix and then use your hands to bring it together into a ball. Allow to rest for 5 minutes.

Briefly knead the dough in the bowl until you achieve a smooth consistency. Dough too wet? Add a little more masa harina flour. Dough too dry? Add a little more water. Divide the dough into 12 pieces, each about 45g / 1¾oz, and roll into balls. If you'd prefer smaller, taco-sized tortillas, each ball should be 35g / 1¼oz.

If using a tortilla press, open it and lay one sheet of non-stick baking parchment over the base of the press. Place your ball in the middle and place another sheet of baking parchment over the top of the ball. Close the lid and press down until the ball has spread. Peel off the parchment. If the edges of your dough are really cracked, you may need to add a little more water to your dough for the next one.

If you don't have a tortilla press, simply place your dough ball on a square sheet of non-stick baking parchment, laid out on a flat surface. Place another square sheet of baking parchment on top and use a heavy ovenproof dish or skillet to flatten it until 3mm / ⅛in thick. Peel off the baking parchment.

Heat a pan over a medium-high heat. Once heated, carefully transfer your flattened dough to the pan. Cook for 30 seconds and then flip. Continue to cook for another 60–90 seconds, then flip back over once more, briefly press down with the spatula and cook for a final 30 seconds – this encourages the tortillas to puff up. Remove from the pan and repeat until you're left with a stack of corn tortilla wraps.

Serve up alongside my one-pot BBQ pulled pork (page 125) or your favourite Mexican food. Or allow them to get a little stale, cut into triangles and fry in oil to make nachos.

TIP:
Don't try this with any other flour, like cornflour (cornstarch); it must be masa harina or it won't work. See the gluten-free store cupboard ingredients chapter on page 12 for more info on this magical flour!

2-INGREDIENT

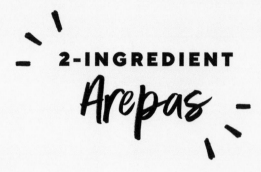

Arepas

MAKES · 8

TAKES · 20 MINUTES

- 300g / 2 cups pre-cooked cornmeal flour (yellow or white)
- 1 tsp salt
- 500ml / 2 cups warm water
- Vegetable oil, for cooking

I had my first arepa at a food market in London and I'm now addicted to making them at home. You essentially use them like a taco, but they're not only crisp on the outside, they're soft and fluffy in the middle and have a wonderful flavour. Cut each one in half and fill with all your favourite Mexican-style fillings. You can easily order pre-cooked cornmeal online and, trust me, you'll be glad you did!

In a large mixing bowl, combine the cornmeal flour and salt. Add the warm water, mix and then use your hands to bring it together into a ball. Allow to rest for 5 minutes.

Briefly knead the dough in the bowl until you achieve a smooth consistency. Dough too wet? Add a little more cornmeal. Dough too dry? Add a little more water.

Divide the dough into 8 portions and roll into large golf balls, around 100g / 3½oz each. One at a time, flatten the balls using your hands to form a flat disc just over 1cm / ½in thick and around 10cm / 4in in diameter. Make sure you don't leave lots of finger indentations in the dough as they won't cook evenly in the pan.

Place a large pan over a medium heat and cover the base with vegetable oil. Once heated, place as many dough discs as will comfortably fit into your pan. Cook for 5 minutes on each side until golden brown. Allow to drain on some kitchen paper and pat dry, then cool for 15 minutes. Repeat until you've used up all your dough.

Slice just over halfway through each arepa with a serrated knife and fill with your favourite Mexican-style fillings. I'd recommend guacamole, fresh salsa and my one-pot pulled pork on page 125.

Store the unfilled arepas in the fridge for up to 5 days and simply bake in the oven to refresh them before enjoying.

TIP:
Don't try this with any other flour, like cornflour (cornstarch); it must be pre-cooked cornmeal flour (see page 12) or it won't work! Please note that pre-cooked cornmeal is different to masa harina flour used in my corn tortilla wraps.

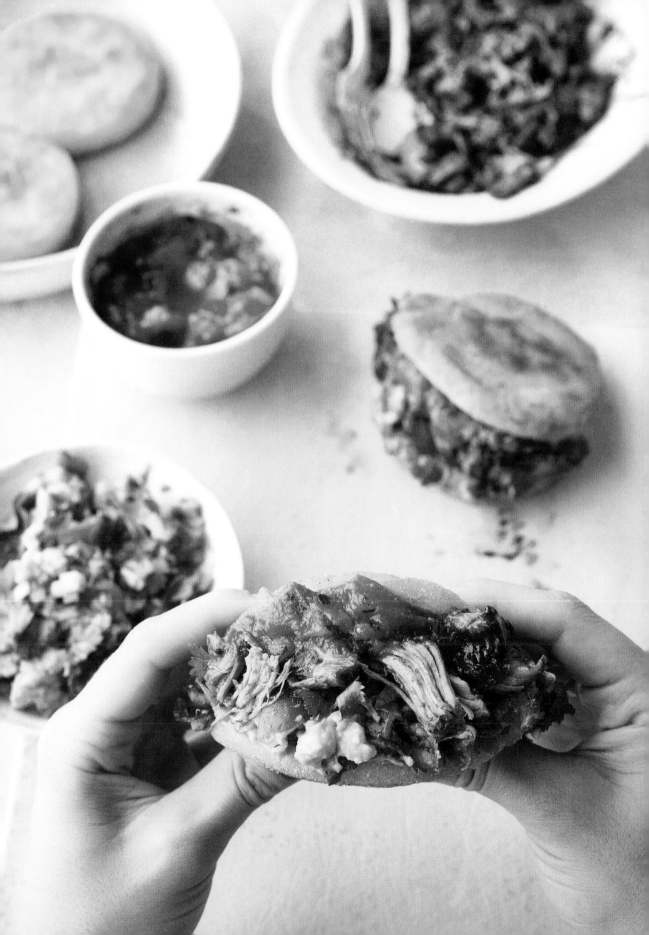

Breakfast and brunch

Whenever I go out for breakfast or brunch, I'm forever confined to a tiny section of the menu. And that's if I'm lucky!

So in this chapter, I decided to create my dream breakfast and brunch menu. There's everything from thick, fluffy banana pancakes, to Belgian waffles and delicious savoury galettes that you absolutely must try.

Of course, I unequivocally had to throw in a few easy, on-the-go options for all those times where we're inevitably in a rush to leave the house. After all, breakfast is the most important meal of the day... especially when you're gluten-free and you can't just buy anything when you're out and about!

3-Ingredient CRÊPES

 use dairy-free milk

 use lactose-free milk

 use lactose-free milk

SERVES · 2 (MAKES 5–6)

TAKES · 15 MINUTES

- 110g / generous ¾ cup gluten-free plain (all-purpose) flour
- 2 large eggs
- 230ml / scant 1 cup milk
- Vegetable oil, for cooking

I thought I'd never eat a crêpe ever again, but actually, they couldn't be any simpler to make. Nobody would ever know they're gluten-free either, so no need to make a separate batch just for yourself. Remember, the thinner you get them, the better!

Grab a large mixing bowl and add your flour. Crack in the eggs and whisk together until smooth. Gradually pour in your milk, while whisking, until you have a lovely, pourable pancake batter. It should be the thickness of a thin cream and not as thin as water. Pour the batter into a jug (pitcher) so it's easier to pour into the pan.

Heat a large frying pan or crêpe pan over a medium heat. Add 1 teaspoon of vegetable oil and brush it over the base of the pan. Once heated, pour the batter into the centre of your pan. Lift the pan and use a circular tilting motion to help the batter spread as much as possible.

Fry for about 1 minute or until the edges are starting to look cooked, then flip and cook for a further 20–30 seconds. Repeat until you've used up all of your batter, adding a teaspoon of oil to the pan per crêpe.

Serve up with toppings of your choice. I love Nutella and ripe bananas, or lemon and brown sugar. Fold them or roll them, it's up to you!

Pictured on page 66

5-INGREDIENT
Banana Pancakes

 use dairy-free milk for batter and oil for frying

 use lactose-free milk

 use lactose-free milk for batter and oil for frying

SERVES · 3 (MAKES 10)

TAKES · 20 MINUTES

- 200g / 1½ cups gluten-free self-raising (self-rising) flour
- 1 tsp gluten-free baking powder
- 300ml / 1¼ cups milk
- 1 large egg
- Vegetable oil or melted butter, for cooking
- 1 ripe banana, cut into slices about 5mm / ¼in thick
- Maple syrup, to serve

Here's a 5-ingredient wonder that only needs a little added oil or butter for frying. These pancakes are thick and fluffy in the middle with caramelized banana in every bite. The only sugar from this recipe comes from the banana, so make sure they're ripe and optionally serve up with maple syrup.

In a mixing bowl, combine the flour and baking powder. In a jug (pitcher), beat together the milk and egg. Create a well in the flour, then pour in the egg and milk mixture, whisking thoroughly for 30 seconds until smooth, like thick cream. Allow the batter to rest for 5–10 minutes.

Heat 1 tablespoon of oil or butter in a frying pan on a medium-low heat. Brush the oil or butter over the base of the pan and, once heated, ladle in one measure of your pancake batter per pancake, about 55g / ¼ cup - you should fit two in the pan at the same time. Immediately place 3–4 slices of banana on each pancake. Placing one slice right in the middle means it'll cook a little quicker!

Cook for 1 minute and, when the edges of the pancakes are looking cooked and the underside is golden, flip over and cook for a further minute before tipping out of the pan. Repeat until all the mixture is used up. Stack up and serve with maple syrup.

TIP:
Looking for American-style gluten-free pancakes? Simply leave out the banana. Alternatively, replace the banana with blueberries for 5-ingredient blueberry pancakes.

Pictured on page 67

Making it vegan?
Use the dairy-free milk of your choice and replace the egg with ½ a ripe banana, mashed. Use oil instead of butter for frying.

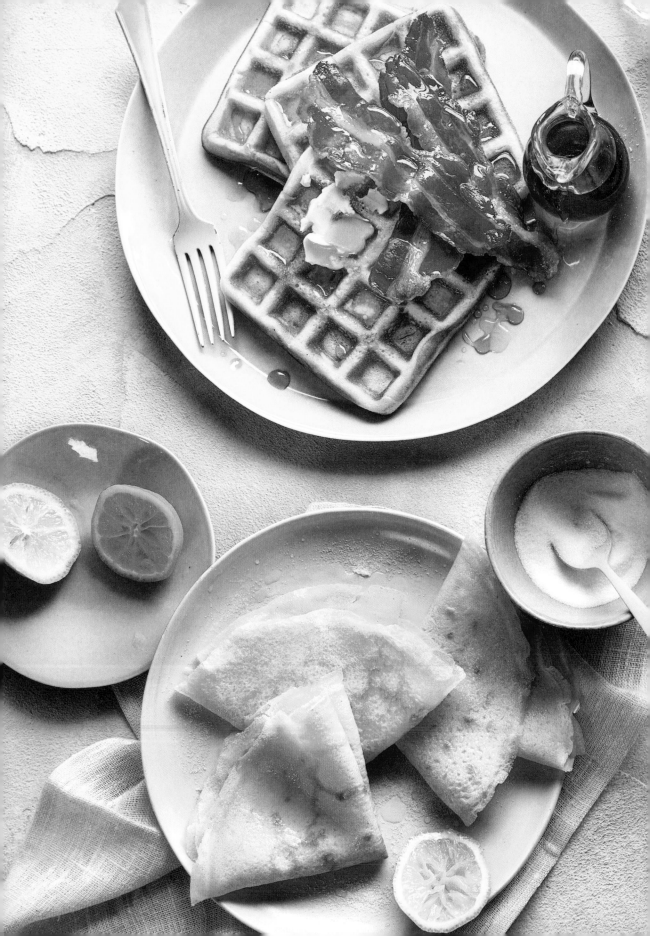

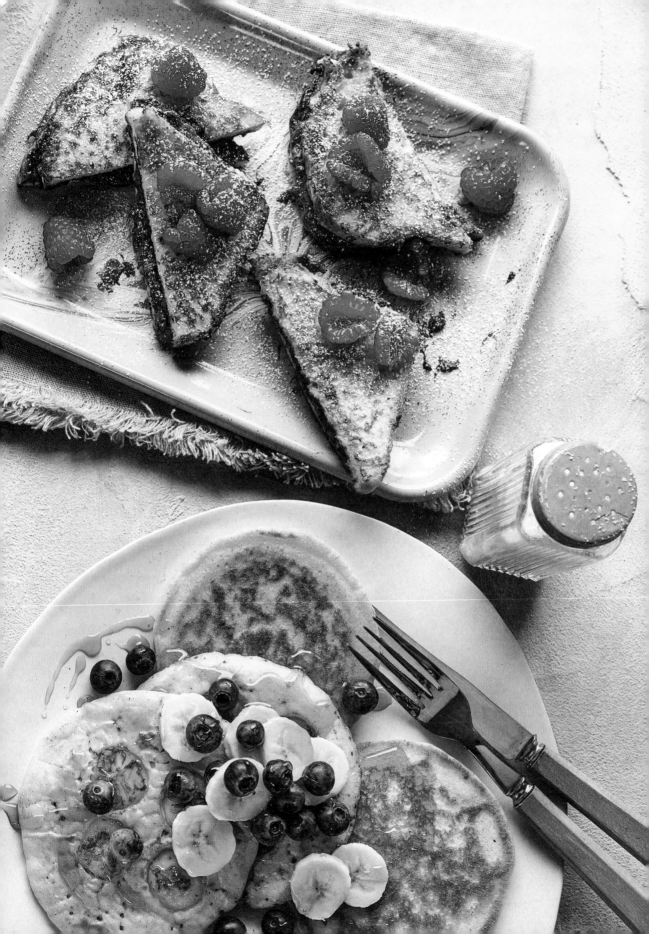

5-INGREDIENT
Chocolate Hazelnut
FRENCH TOAST

SERVES · 2

TAKES · 10 MINUTES

- 4 slices of gluten-free bread
- 4 tbsp chocolate hazelnut spread
- 75ml / ⅓ cup milk
- 2 eggs
- 15g / 1 tbsp butter

To serve (optional)

- Icing (confectioners') sugar
- Maple syrup
- Fresh raspberries

This is my go-to weekend breakfast after a long week. With gooey chocolate hazelnut spread in between two slices of golden, gluten-free French toast, I'm sure it's easy to imagine why!

Take your bread and chocolate hazelnut spread and make two sandwiches. No need to cut them in half.

Grab a large mixing bowl and add your milk and eggs. Beat until smooth.

Dunk your sandwiches into the egg mixture until both sides are as soggy as possible. Don't forget the edges of the sandwich too! Allow them both to soak in the mixture for a few minutes.

Add your butter to a large frying pan and place over a medium heat. Once the butter has melted, add both sandwiches and fry on both sides for 2–3 minutes or until golden brown. Remove from the pan and place onto a plate. Dust with icing sugar and serve up with maple syrup and raspberries, if you like.

TIP:
This also works really well using jam (jelly) instead of chocolate hazelnut spread.

Pictured on page 67

Making it dairy-free?
Use dairy-free milk and a dairy-free butter alternative. Ensure you use a dairy-free chocolate hazelnut spread.

Making it low lactose?
Use lactose-free milk. Ensure you use a lactose-free chocolate hazelnut spread.

Making it low FODMAP?
Use lactose-free milk. Ensure you use a low FODMAP chocolate hazelnut spread.

Making it vegan?
Follow the advice above to make this dairy-free. Then substitute the eggs for 1 tbsp ground flaxseed. Once added, allow the mixture to rest for 5 minutes.

6-INGREDIENT
Belgian Waffles

 use dairy-free milk

 use lactose-free milk

**SERVES · 2
(MAKES 6 WAFFLES)**

TAKES · 15 MINUTES

- 150g / 1 cup plus 2 tbsp gluten-free self-raising (self-rising) flour
- 3 tbsp caster (superfine) sugar
- ½ tsp gluten-free baking powder
- 250ml / 1 cup milk
- 1 egg
- 2 tsp vanilla extract
- Vegetable oil, for cooking (if needed)
- Maple syrup, to serve

Spoiler alert: you can only make waffles if you have a waffle maker. But as literally nowhere that sells waffles will _ever_ have a separate 'gluten-free only' waffle maker, it sort of makes sense that you have one instead, right? These waffles are lovely and crisp on the outside, soft and fluffy in the middle with a subtle, sweet vanilla flavour. Pass me the maple syrup please.

In a large mixing bowl, combine the flour, sugar and baking powder. In a jug (pitcher), beat together the milk, egg and vanilla. Create a well in the flour and pour in the milk and egg mixture, whisking thoroughly for 30 seconds until nice and smooth. Allow the batter to rest for 5–10 minutes.

While your batter is resting, start heating up your waffle maker. All waffle makers vary, so follow the instructions of your particular machine. If yours requests that you brush a little vegetable oil onto it first, make sure you do this once it's heated.

Once your waffle maker has heated, pour in one measure of your batter, about 55g / ¼ cup at a time, and close the lid. Cook for 3–4 minutes until consistently golden on the outside (different models will vary). Once cooked, remove and keep warm in a low oven while you use up the rest of your batter.

Serve up with maple syrup and whatever you like on top. For brunch, I love fresh blueberries and Mark loves crispy, smoky bacon with maple syrup. Or you can go wild and serve it with my gluten-free KFC (page 117) on top.

TIP:
If your waffles keep sticking to the waffle maker, brush it with a little oil before you pour in your batter. My waffle maker is non-stick so I don't really need to, but we also have a cast-iron waffle maker where this step is essential.

Pictured on page 66

Making it vegan?
Use the dairy-free milk of your choice and replace the egg with half a mashed ripe banana.

MAPLE, PECAN, DARK CHOCOLATE OR STRAWBERRY
Granola

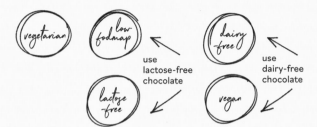

vegetarian

low fodmap → use lactose-free chocolate

dairy free → use dairy-free chocolate

lactose free ↙

vegan ↙

MAKES · 500G / 18OZ (10 SERVINGS)

TAKES · 20 MINUTES

For the granola base
- 150ml / ⅝ cup maple syrup
- 1 tsp ground cinnamon
- ½ tsp vanilla extract
- 50ml / 3½ tbsp vegetable oil
- 200g / 2 cups gluten-free oats
- 100g / 4 cups gluten-free puffed rice cereal
- 40g / ½ cup desiccated (dried shredded) coconut
- Pinch of salt

For maple pecan granola
- 75g / ¾ cup pecans, chopped
- 30g / ⅓ cup flaked (slivered) almonds

For dark chocolate granola
- 100g / 3½oz 50% or 70% dark chocolate, roughly chopped

For strawberry granola
- 12g / ½oz freeze-dried strawberries

For muggles, there's literally an entire aisle dedicated to boatloads of different breakfast cereals. On the other hand, we only get the choice of five if we're lucky. So I decided to recreate all those lovely variations of granola that I can never eat – choose whichever flavour you want!

Preheat the oven to 170°C fan / 190°C / 375°F and line two baking trays with non-stick baking parchment.

Grab a large mixing bowl and add the maple syrup, cinnamon, vanilla and oil. Mix until well combined. Next, add the oats, puffed rice cereal, coconut and salt. Give it all a good stir until everything is evenly mixed and coated, then pour the mixture onto the two baking trays and spread out evenly.

Pop both trays into the preheated oven for 15 minutes or until everything is golden brown, turning the granola over halfway through. If making the maple pecan version of this recipe, add in your chopped pecans and flaked almonds halfway through the cooking time too.

If making the dark chocolate or strawberry version of this recipe, allow the granola to fully cool before mixing in your chocolate or strawberries.

Pop into an airtight container and store for up to a month. Enjoy with plain yoghurt or milk.

TIP:
This recipe contains gluten-free oats; check page 12 for more info on them if you can't find them where you live.

Blueberry and Banana
BAKED PORRIDGE

 use dairy-free yoghurt

 use lactose-free yoghurt

 use lactose-free yoghurt

SERVES · 3

TAKES · 35 MINUTES

- 100g / 1 cup gluten-free oats
- 300g / 1½ cups plain yoghurt
- 3 eggs
- 1 tbsp maple syrup, plus extra to serve
- 1 tsp ground cinnamon
- 1 ripe banana, chopped into chunks
- 100g / ¾ cup blueberries, frozen or fresh

To serve

- Strawberries, sliced (optional)
- Crunchy peanut butter (optional)

Meet the zero-effort breakfast I'd happily eat for dessert. Packed with sticky gluten-free oats, bursting blueberries, chunks of gooey banana and a hint of cinnamon, this is the ultimate way to start the day.

Preheat the oven to 180°C fan / 200°C / 400°F.

Place all the ingredients (reserving a few blueberries for the top) in a large mixing bowl and stir until everything is thoroughly combined.

Pour the mixture into an ovenproof dish and top with the reserved blueberries. You can either make one big batch or smaller, individual portions, depending on the size of your dish.

Cook in the oven for 30–35 minutes, then remove from the oven and serve warm. Optionally top with sliced strawberries, a dollop of peanut butter and some maple syrup.

TIP:
If you can't find or tolerate gluten-free oats, rice flake porridge also works really well here.

Making it vegan?
Instead of using eggs, add 1 large mashed banana. Use dairy-free yoghurt.

6-INGREDIENT
Breakfast Bars

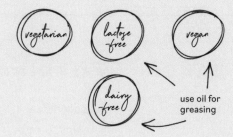

vegetarian lactose free vegan

dairy free

use oil for greasing

MAKES · 9

TAKES · 20 MINUTES

- Butter or oil, for greasing
- 4 ripe bananas (around 460g / 15oz peeled weight)
- 120g / generous ½ cup peanut butter (smooth or crunchy)
- 250g / 2½ cups gluten-free oats
- 60g / ½ cup dried cranberries
- 60g / ½ cup pecans, chopped
- 30g / ¼ cup pumpkin seeds

What can I say? These bars are stupidly easy and quick to make, packed with tons of goodness and they taste divine. Every bite is bursting with banana flavour, a hint of peanut butter and a welcome sweetness from the cranberries. The nuts and seeds add a lovely crunch too. This is my go-to on-the-go gluten-free breakfast!

Preheat the oven to 160°C fan / 180°C / 350°F. Lightly grease a 20cm / 8in square baking tin (pan) and line with non-stick baking parchment.

Mash your bananas in a large mixing bowl until nice and smooth, then mix in your peanut butter. Stir in your oats until well combined. Mix in your dried cranberries, pecans and pumpkin seeds, reserving a few of the pumpkin seeds to scatter on top.

Spread the mixture into your tin and evenly compact it in. Try to get it nice and level on top before scattering on your extra pumpkin seeds. Lightly compact those in too, using the back of a fork.

Bake in the oven for around 15 minutes, then remove and allow to cool before cutting into bars.

TIP:
You can also substitute the peanut butter with chocolate hazelnut spread if you're not a huge PB fan.

This recipe contains gluten-free oats; check page 12 for more info on them if you can't find them where you live.

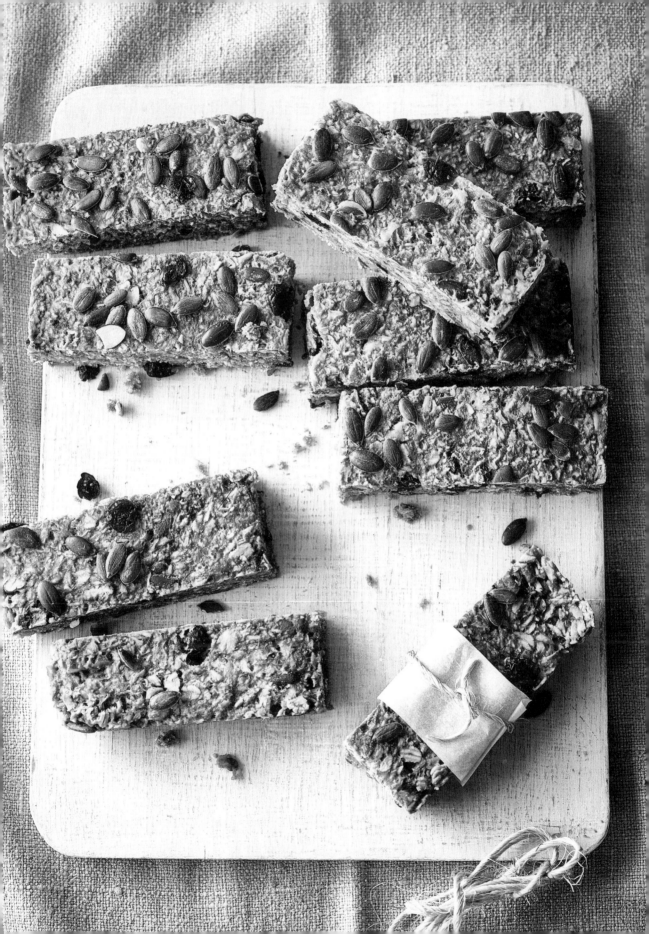

HAM AND CHEESE
Breakfast Galettes

dairy-free — use dairy-free cheese for filling and oil for frying

low fodmap

vegetarian — replace the ham with wilted spinach

low lactose

MAKES · 3

TAKES · 20 MINUTES

- 80g / ⅔ cup gluten-free buckwheat flour
- ¼ tsp salt
- 1 egg
- 250ml / 1 cup water
- 3 tsp butter (or oil), for cooking
- Black pepper

For the filling

- 3 eggs
- 75g / 3oz hard cheese, grated (I recommend Comté)
- 6 slices of thick-cut ham

Galettes are traditionally made with buckwheat flour, but make sure yours is gluten-free. These are just like the galettes I had in Paris - thin and crisp, filled with an egg with runny yolk, melted cheese and ham. It's the perfect easy breakfast or brunch.

Add the buckwheat flour, salt, egg and water to a large mixing bowl and mix together using a fork, until you have a smooth batter. Allow to rest for 10 minutes.

Heat a large frying pan or crêpe pan over a high heat. Add 1 teaspoon of the butter and spread around so that the base of the pan is covered. Pour in enough batter to cover two-thirds of the base of the pan, then lift the pan and use a circular tilting motion to help the batter spread to the remaining third of the pan. This will help ensure a perfectly thin and crispy galette.

Allow to cook for 15–20 seconds, then reduce down to a medium heat. Crack an egg into the middle of the galette and, using a fork, carefully spread the egg white so it covers as much of the galette as possible.

Sprinkle a third of the cheese all over the egg white and place two small slices of ham either side of the yolk. Fold the edges in using a small palette knife so that it forms a square, and cook for 2–3 minutes.

Season with a little black pepper, and transfer to a plate (serve with fresh rocket / arugula on the side). Repeat until all of your galette batter has been used, remembering to adjust the heat back to high for the start of each galette.

TIP:
Using butter to fry your galettes gives them tons of flavour!

Making it vegan?
Mixing 100g / ⅘ cup gluten-free buckwheat flour with 250ml / 1 cup water (leaving out the egg) will make lovely vegan galette batter that you can fill with whatever you like. Use oil instead of butter for frying.

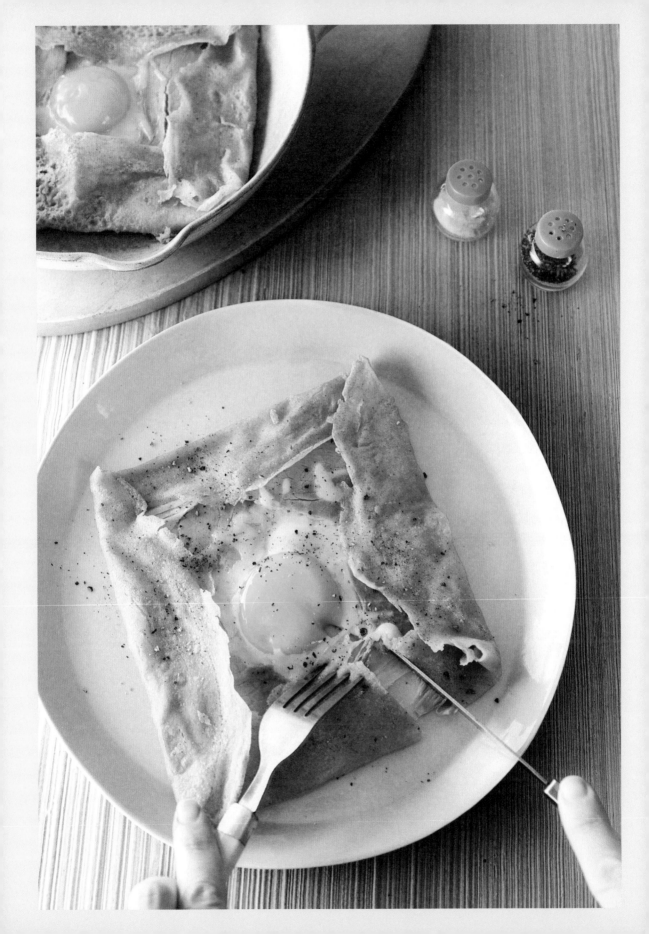

Courgette and Halloumi
MUFFINS

 use lactose-free milk

 use lactose-free milk

MAKES · 10–12

TAKES · 30 MINUTES

- 60ml / ¼ cup olive oil, plus extra for greasing
- 1 egg
- 200ml / generous ¾ cup milk
- 250g / generous 1¾ cups gluten-free self-raising (self-rising) flour
- 2 tsp gluten-free baking powder
- 150g / 5¼oz halloumi cheese, grated, plus a little extra (optional) to finish
- 2 tbsp dried mixed herbs
- Handful of fresh chives, chopped
- 1 courgette (zucchini), grated
- Sweet chilli sauce, to serve (optional)

If you're a massive halloumi fan like I am, you'll absolutely love these on-the-go brunch muffins. They're cheesy and herby, with a light, soft middle and a crisp exterior.

Preheat the oven to 200°C fan / 220°C / 425°F. Grease the holes of a muffin tray with a little vegetable oil.

Grab a mixing bowl and add the oil, egg and milk, whisking until well combined. Add in the flour and baking powder along with your grated halloumi, mixed herbs, chives and courgette. Stir everything until there are no visible lumps of flour left, then stop: definitely don't over mix this one!

Divide the mixture equally between the holes of the muffin tray and cook in the oven for 20 minutes, then remove the muffins from the tray by gently easing them out with a small palette knife. Allow to cool on a wire rack.

Once cooled, dollop a little sweet chilli sauce on top and garnish with a small slice of griddled or lightly fried halloumi, if you like.

Making it dairy-free?
Use dairy-free milk and good dairy-free cheese that melts well.

Making it vegan?
Follow the advice above to make it dairy-free and replace the egg with 3 tbsp aquafaba (whisked until frothy).

·HASH BROWN·
Breakfast cups

 use dairy-free cheese and a dairy-free butter alternative

 leave out the bacon

MAKES · 9

TAKES · 45 MINUTES

- 500g / 18oz potatoes
- 80g / 3oz extra mature Cheddar cheese, grated
- 60g / 4 tbsp butter, melted
- ½ tsp salt
- 9 small eggs
- 50g / 3½oz smoky bacon, finely diced
- Handful of fresh chives, chopped, to serve

This breakfast hero is everything I love about a full-English breakfast in one glorious yet humble little cup. Imagine a crispy hash brown filled with baked eggs and topped with crispy bacon. Enjoy at home or on-the-go, hot or cold. They even make great party food canapés too.

Preheat the oven to 180°C fan / 200°C / 400°F.

Peel your potatoes, grate them on the coarse side of a box grater, and transfer to a sieve. Place the sieve under cold running water to wash off all the sticky, starchy residue, then squeeze out the potato by hand to remove as much moisture as possible. Place on kitchen paper and allow to dry for 10 minutes.

Grab a large mixing bowl and add the grated potato to it, along with the cheese, melted butter and salt. Mix it all together so everything is nicely combined.

Grab a muffin tray and add one modest tablespoon of your hash brown mixture to 9 of the holes. Use your fingers to compress it in and form a thin base for each hash brown cup. Add another tablespoon on top of each hash brown base and compress it up the sides of each muffin hole, making sure the sides aren't too thin at the top or they'll brown too quickly.

Cook in the oven for 15 minutes, then crack an egg into each hole and top with some bacon. Place back in the oven for 10 minutes, then remove and allow to cool briefly before topping with the chives. Dip them in ketchup and thank me later!

STARTERS, SIDES AND SNACKS

This chapter is my 'greatest hits' of all the awesome starters, sides and snacks that I can never order when I'm eating out. Too often, out of an entire list of sides and starters, the only thing that's gluten-free is a side salad. And that's definitely not OK!

So here's how to create everything from prawn toast and spring rolls, to veggie samosas, calamari, triple cheese doughballs and even Yorkshire puddings.

I also had to throw in a couple of classic British snacks that we always miss out on. So let's reclaim starters, sides and snacks!

SESAME
Prawn Toast

   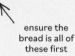

ensure the bread is all of these first

SERVES · 5–6
(MAKES 24–36 PIECES)

TAKES · 30 MINUTES

- 6–9 slices of white gluten-free bread (page 41 or store-bought)
- 70g / ½ cup sesame seeds
- 150ml / ⅝ cup vegetable oil

For the prawn paste

- 165g / 6oz raw shelled and deveined prawns (shrimp)
- 1 tsp minced ginger paste
- ¼ tsp caster (superfine) sugar
- ¼ tsp black pepper
- 2 tbsp water
- 1 tbsp gluten-free soy sauce
- Pinch of salt

Who'd have thought that something I missed out on for years was so easy to make gluten-free? I figured out a way to make these without deep-frying them, but they still taste *exactly* the same – golden, crispy with that lovely prawn and sesame combo. I often make a big batch and freeze them for our future fakeaway nights.

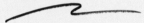

Preheat the oven to 200°C fan / 220°C / 425°F.

Place the ingredients for your prawn paste in a food processor and blitz to a smooth, spreadable consistency. If you don't have a food processor, use a sharp knife to chop the prawns into a smooth paste – this can take a while so be patient! Ensure they're not chunky and are as mushy as possible. Then place them in a bowl, add the rest of the prawn paste ingredients and mix until well combined.

Spread this mixture across each slice of bread, making sure you go right up to the edges. You should have enough prawn mixture for up to 9 slices of bread if you're economical with your spreading.

Pour your sesame seeds onto a large plate and spread them out evenly. Place your bread prawn-side down in the sesame seeds until fully covered. Repeat for all the slices of bread, then cut each slice into 4 triangles.

Pour your vegetable oil into a small bowl. Dip each prawn toast triangle into the oil until fully submerged. Then place them all on a baking tray and cook in the oven for 8–10 minutes until lightly golden brown, flipping them over halfway through.

Serve up with your favourite gluten-free sweet chilli dipping sauce.

TIP:
You can also freeze your raw prawn toast after dipping them in oil. Then when you want to eat them, just cook straight from frozen for 12–14 minutes.

Pictured on page 83

Making it veggie? Or vegan?
Ensure you bread is veggie/vegan. Replace the prawns with the same weight of mushrooms and continue the recipe as directed.

Crispy Chicken
SPRING ROLLS

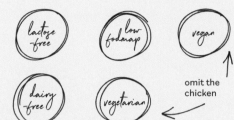

lactose-free   low fodmap   vegan

dairy-free   vegetarian

omit the chicken

MAKES · 15

TAKES · 45 MINUTES

- 125g / 4½oz chicken breast fillets
- ½ carrot
- ½ red (bell) pepper
- 60g / 2oz green cabbage
- Handful of spring onion (scallion) greens
- 2 tbsp garlic-infused oil
- 1 tbsp gluten-free soy sauce
- 1 tsp sesame oil
- 50g / ½ cup beansprouts
- 15 rice paper spring roll wrappers
- 500ml / 2 cups vegetable oil

With a crispy exterior that conceals tons of tender chicken and perfectly cooked veg, one spring roll is never enough! Rice paper spring roll wrappers are naturally gluten-free, and making crispy spring rolls with them is incredibly simple. You can replace the chicken with my crispy duck recipe on page 111, for crispy duck spring rolls.

Thinly slice your chicken, then chop each slice into small strips – no big chunks of chicken here please! Slice your carrot and red pepper into long, thin strips. Shred your cabbage using a mandoline or chop using a sharp knife. Slice your spring onion greens into thin strips.

Place a wok over a medium heat and add your garlic-infused oil. Add your chicken strips and stir-fry for 1 minute, then add in the carrot, red pepper and cabbage and stir-fry for 2–3 minutes. Add in the soy sauce and sesame oil as well as the beansprouts and spring onion. Continue to stir-fry until the beansprouts soften a little. Remove from the heat and allow to cool completely.

Time to construct your spring rolls – the fun part! Add some warm water to a large lipped plate so it's nice and shallow. Take one sheet of rice paper and dip it in for 5 seconds, immersing it completely. Then place the wrapper on a wooden surface or a damp cloth. After around 10–15 seconds, the rice paper should no longer feel plasticky and hard; it should feel more flexible and slightly sticky.

Add 1 tablespoon of the filling to your rice paper, placing it in a line, just below the middle of the rice wrapper. Make sure you get a few bits of chicken into each spring roll. Fold the bottom of the rice wrapper so that it just overlaps the filling. Fold in the left and right sides of the wrapper. Now you're ready to roll!

Tightly roll it forwards so that you create a small spring roll about 6–7cm / 2½–2¾in long. Repeat until you've used all your filling. Don't let your constructed spring rolls touch each other or they'll stick together.

At this point, you've basically created Vietnamese summer rolls and you can actually eat them just like that! But if you want *crispy* spring rolls, keep following the recipe.

In a (clean) wok, pour in your vegetable oil so it is about 2cm / ¾in deep. Place over a medium heat for 8–10 minutes or until it reaches 170°C / 340°F – test with a cooking thermometer, or by using the wooden spoon handle test (page 19).

In batches, carefully lower your spring rolls into the oil, making sure they aren't touching each other – they should sizzle nicely. Cook for around 5 minutes, turning halfway through, until slightly golden and crispy, then remove from the oil and place onto a wire rack set over a baking tray to drain.

Serve up with your favourite gluten-free sweet chilli dipping sauce.

TIP:
Bigger spring rolls won't be as crisp after cooking, so make sure they're no more than 7cm / 2¾in long.

Pictured on page 83

STICKY CHINESE-STYLE
Spare Ribs

ensure five
spice is onion/
garlic-free

SERVES · 4

TAKES · 30 MINUTES

- 1 tbsp garlic-infused oil
- 500g / 18oz pork ribs, cut into 7.5cm / 3in long chunks

For the sauce

- 2 tsp Chinese five spice
- 1 tbsp dry sherry
- 3 tbsp gluten-free soy sauce (or gluten-free dark soy sauce, page 35)
- 3 tbsp white rice vinegar
- 4 tbsp light brown sugar
- 50ml / 3½ tbsp water

Yep, all the sides are back on the menu! These are sticky and sweet with tons of tender pork that falls off the bone. So often, recipes like this call for Shaoxing rice wine vinegar, but it actually contains wheat, so I simply use dry sherry instead. You can save on preparation of your pork ribs when you're still at the shops, by buying meaty pork ribs that have already been cut to the right length – just ask the butcher! I say this because they're impossible to chop at home unless you have a large meat cleaver.

In a small bowl, combine all the ingredients for your sauce and mix well.

Grab a Dutch oven or a large lidded flameproof casserole dish and add the garlic-infused oil. Place over a medium heat, add your pork rib chunks and lightly fry all sides for 2–3 minutes.

Add your sauce and bring to the boil, then turn the heat down as low as possible and pop the lid on. Cook for 20–25 minutes, turning the ribs every 7–8 minutes or so. Remove the lid, turn up to a medium heat and simmer until the sauce reduces and becomes nice and sticky. Once reduced, continue to cook until the pork ribs brown a little.

Serve alongside all your Chinese takeaway favourites in the Fakeaways chapter, pages 101–125.

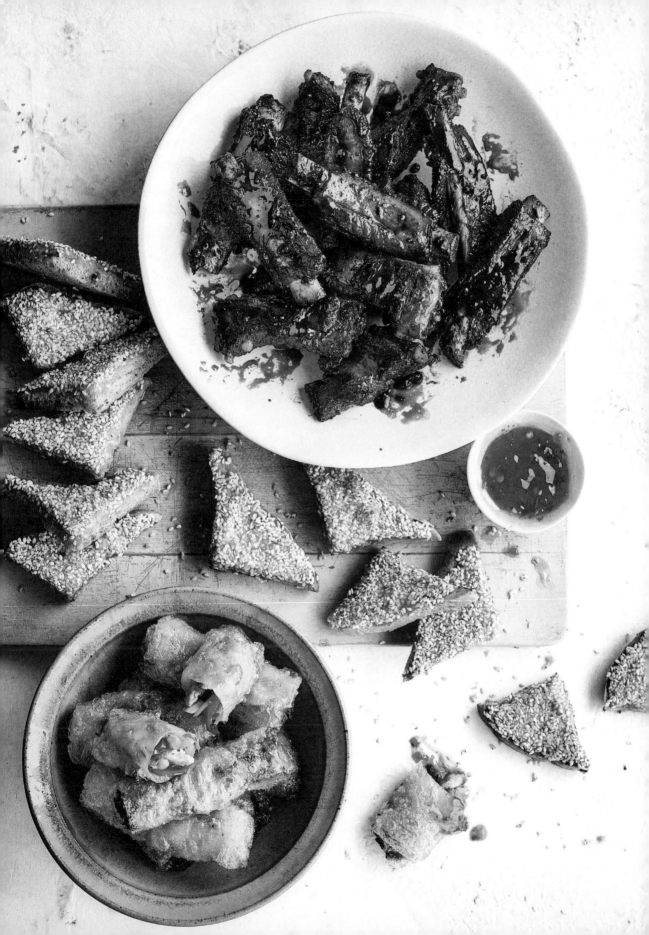

OVEN-BAKED *Bhajis*

ensure curry powder is onion/garlic-free and use gf plain flour

MAKES · 12

TAKES · 40 MINUTES

- 450g / 1lb courgettes (zucchini)
- 100g / ¾ cup gluten-free plain (all-purpose) flour or gram (chickpea) flour
- ½ tsp mild curry powder
- 1 tsp ground cumin
- 1 tsp dried chilli flakes
- Pinch of ground turmeric
- 1 tsp minced ginger paste
- Handful of fresh chives, chopped
- 3 eggs
- 4 tbsp garlic-infused oil

These bhajis are lovely and crisp, mildly spicy and perfect alongside all your favourite curries. Using a muffin tray makes them considerably less messy to make and there's no deep-frying required.

Preheat the oven to 180°C fan / 200°C / 400°F.

Chop your courgettes into strips that are 4mm / ⅛in thick, 4mm / ⅛in wide and about 6cm / 2½in long. The thinner and more uniform in size your strips are, the quicker and more consistently they'll cook.

Put your courgette strips into a large mixing bowl. Throw in your flour, spices, ginger paste and chives. Give it a good mix and crack in the eggs. Mix once more until all the courgette is evenly coated.

Grab a muffin tray. Add 1 teaspoon of garlic-infused oil to each hole. Then, using a tablespoon, spoon your courgette mixture into each muffin hole until each one is evenly filled. Using your fingers, make sure that there are not too many bits of courgette sticking up into the air as these will burn.

Cook in the oven for 30 minutes, then remove and use a spoon to ease them out of their holes. Serve up with mint raita alongside your favourite curries and my gluten-free Peshwari naan breads (page 57) or gluten-free veggie samosas (opposite).

TIP:
Feel free to use onion instead of courgette for these, but trust me, courgette works wonders and soaks up all that lovely flavour!

Making it vegan?
Simply replace the eggs with 9 tbsp aquafaba (whisked until frothy).

Cheat's
VEGETABLE SAMOSAS

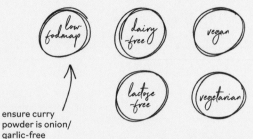

ensure curry powder is onion/garlic-free

MAKES · 10

TAKES · 45–50 MINUTES

- 5 gluten-free tortilla wraps (page 59 or store-bought)
- Vegetable oil, for cooking

For the filling

- 1 potato, peeled
- 1 carrot, peeled
- 3 tbsp garlic-infused oil
- 50g / scant ½ cup frozen peas
- 1½ tsp mild curry powder
- ¼ tsp dried chilli flakes
- 1 tsp smoked paprika
- Handful of spring onion (scallion) greens, chopped
- Handful of coriander (cilantro), chopped
- Salt

For the 'glue'

- 2 tbsp gluten-free plain (all-purpose) flour
- 3 tbsp water

These samosas are super crisp on the outside and crammed with tons of warming, mildly spicy veg in the middle. Using gluten-free tortilla wraps is a great little hack to skip having to make your own dough. Either bake these in the oven, or deep-fry them – it's up to you!

Place your peeled, whole potato and carrot in a saucepan. Cover with cold water and place over a medium heat. Bring to the boil and simmer until both are cooked. Drain and allow to cool, then cut into small cubes.

Add your garlic-infused oil to a large pan and place over a medium heat. Add the frozen peas and briefly fry until defrosted. Add in your cooked potato and carrot cubes, then briefly stir so everything is nicely coated in the oil. Add all the spices with salt to taste, then fry for another 2 minutes until fragrant. Stir in your chopped spring onion and coriander and remove the pan from the heat.

In a small dish, mix your flour and water to form a paste, or 'glue'.

Cut one of your tortilla wraps in half using a pizza cutter. Form a tight cone in your hand with both of the straight sides overlapping to form a seam. Using your fingers, dab a little of the 'glue' along the seam of the cone and press together to glue it shut. Make sure you have a nice, sharp point with no hole at the end.

Holding the cone in your hand, spoon in your filling, leaving a 1cm / ½in gap at the top. Dab a little of your 'glue' all along the edge and pinch shut. Make sure you seal it up well so the filling can't escape – add as much 'glue' as you need! Repeat until you've used up all your wraps and filling.

At this point, you can either brush the samosas with vegetable oil and bake on a baking tray in the oven at 180°C fan / 200°C / 400°F for 12 minutes, until nicely browned, turning them over halfway to ensure both sides are nice and crisp. Or you can deep-fry them for the ultimate crispy finish. Half-fill a large, heavy-based saucepan with vegetable oil and place over a medium heat for about 15 minutes, until it reaches 170°C / 340°F – test with a cooking thermometer or by using the wooden spoon handle test (page 19). Then, carefully lower the samosas into the oil in batches and cook for 8 minutes or until golden, turning them halfway.

Serve up alongside your favourite curries and my gluten-free Peshwari naan breads (page 57) or gluten-free bhajis (opposite).

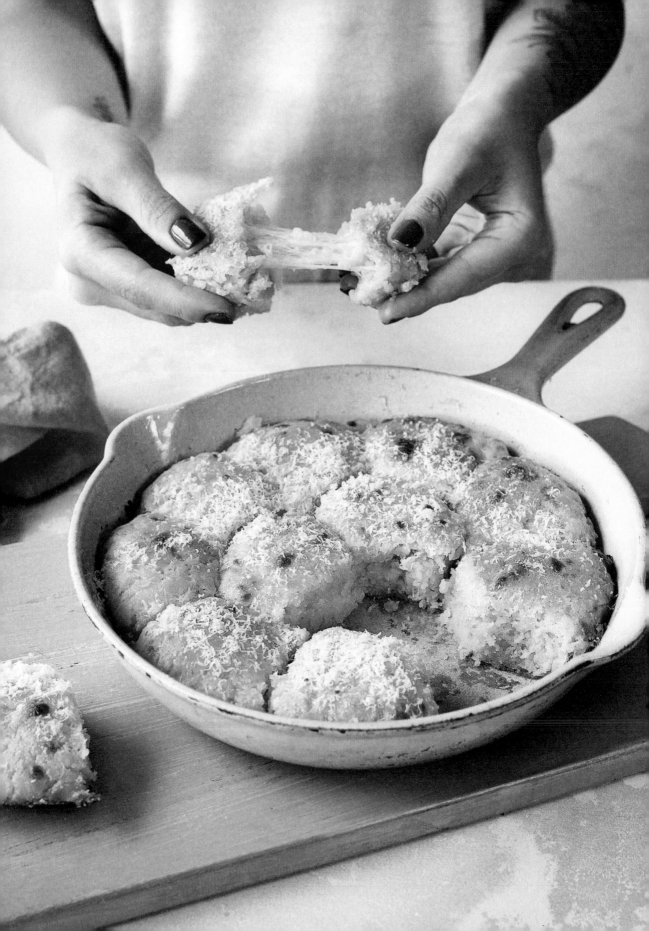

TRIPLE CHEESE
Doughballs

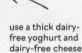 use a thick dairy-free yoghurt and dairy-free cheese

 use lactose-free Greek yoghurt and lactose-free cheese

MAKES · 12

**TAKES · 30 MINUTES
+ 1 HOUR PROVING**

- 75ml / 5 tbsp warm water
- 10g / 1 tbsp caster (superfine) sugar
- 5g / ⅙oz active dried yeast (ensure gluten-free)
- 225g / 1¾ cups gluten-free plain (all-purpose) flour
- ¼ tsp xanthan gum
- ½ tsp salt
- 150g / ⅔ cup Greek yoghurt
- 20ml / 1½ tbsp garlic-infused oil, plus extra for greasing and brushing
- 85g / 3oz extra mature Cheddar cheese, grated
- 150g / 5¼oz mozzarella cheese, chopped into 1.5cm / ½in cubes

For the topping
- 15g / ½oz pecorino cheese, grated
- Salt

My triple cheese doughballs are everything I thought gluten-free doughballs could never be. Packed with stringy mozzarella in the middle, they're crisp on the outside, light and fluffy inside and they tear like real pizza dough. If you didn't know better, you'd think someone accidentally served you gluten-filled doughballs by mistake!

In a jug (pitcher), mix together your warm water, sugar and yeast. Allow to stand for 10 minutes until nice and frothy.

In a large mixing bowl, add your flour, xanthan gum, salt, yoghurt, oil and grated Cheddar cheese, along with the frothy yeast mixture. Mix with a spatula until well combined and a dough forms.

Place your dough in a clean bowl with cling film (plastic wrap) over the top and leave to prove for 1 hour in a warm place, until slightly bigger and feeling a little spongy.

Lightly oil your work surface and turn your dough out onto it. Divide into 12 pieces, each weighing about 45g / 1½oz.

Roll each piece of dough into a ball. Take a ball, flatten it in the palm of your hand and insert a cube of mozzarella into the centre. Gently pull the dough over the mozzarella so it's completely covered and roll it back into a ball. Repeat for all the pieces of dough.

At this point, you can prove the dough a second time (this results in slightly bigger, puffier doughballs) if you like. If doing this, place the doughballs in an ovenproof dish (or skillet) in a cluster, with a 2mm / ¹⁄₁₆in gap between each. Cover with cling film and leave to prove in a warm place for 1 more hour.

If skipping the second prove, place your doughballs in an ovenproof dish (or skillet) in a cluster, ensuring that they're all slightly touching each other. Preheat your oven to 200°C fan / 220°C / 425°F.

Brush the doughballs with a little extra oil and sprinkle with the pecorino and a little salt.

Cook in the oven for 20 minutes until golden on top. A little of the cheese might ooze out, but that's OK! Serve up immediately for hot, stringy, cheesy doughball goodness.

CRISPY Calamari

SERVES · 2

TAKES · 30 MINUTES

- 1.5l / 6½ cups vegetable oil
- 300g / 10½oz cleaned squid (keep the tentacles)
- 50g / 6 tbsp gluten-free plain (all-purpose) flour

For the batter

- 60g / 6½ tbsp gluten-free plain (all-purpose) flour
- 30g / ⅓ cup cornflour (cornstarch)
- 1 tsp gluten-free baking powder
- ¼ tsp salt
- ½ tsp cayenne pepper
- 125ml / ½ cup carbonated water

For the herby dip

- 100ml / scant ⅓ cup mayonnaise
- 1½ tsp garlic-infused oil
- 1½ tsp dried mixed herbs

My calamari is incredibly crisp with a light and airy batter – guaranteed crunch in every bite. Most importantly, the squid inside remains lovely and tender too! Serve it up with my 3-ingredient herby dip and contemplate why you literally never see gluten-free calamari on any menu, ever.

Pour the vegetable oil into a large, heavy-based saucepan, making sure it is no more than half full. Place over a medium heat and heat for about 15 minutes until it reaches 170°C / 340°F – test the temperature with a cooking thermometer or by using the wooden spoon handle test (page 19).

While your oil is heating, cut the squid into 5mm / ¼in rings and pat dry with kitchen paper to remove excess moisture.

Combine all the dry batter ingredients in a large mixing bowl. Mix until consistent, then add your carbonated water and whisk together until smooth and without lumps.

Spread the flour onto a large plate. Take a third of your squid rings/ tentacles and roll them around in the flour until well coated. Once your oil is hot, take a few pieces of your coated squid and dip them into the batter, ensuring they are well coated. Carefully lower into the hot oil. It should calmly bubble as they cook, without excessive spitting.

Cook for 2–3 minutes until nice and golden, giving the tentacles an extra minute or two if they're particularly chunky. Remove with a slotted spoon and transfer to a wire rack set over a baking tray to drain then repeat with the rest of the squid.

Mix together the ingredients for your herby dip and serve immediately.

TIP:
Give the batter a regular mix, as the cornflour will sink to the bottom of the mixture after a few minutes.

Making it vegan? Or veggie?
See opposite for my crispy tempura veg recipe instead. Alternatively, you can use this batter to make your own homemade onion rings. I can't tolerate onion, so enjoy them for me! Don't forget to use vegan mayo for the dip.

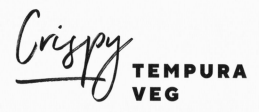

Crispy TEMPURA VEG

SERVES · 4

TAKES · 40 MINUTES

- 1.5l / 6½ cups vegetable oil
- ½ red (bell) pepper
- ½ courgette (zucchini)
- ½ aubergine (eggplant)
- ½ sweet potato, peeled
- 70g / ½ cup gluten-free plain (all-purpose) flour

For the batter

- 90g / ¾ cup gluten-free plain (all-purpose) flour
- 45g / ½ cup cornflour (cornstarch)
- 1½ tsp gluten-free baking powder
- ½ tsp salt
- ½ tsp cayenne pepper
- 185ml / ¾ cup carbonated water

For the dipping sauce

- 3 tbsp gluten-free soy sauce
- 2 tbsp water
- 1 tsp caster (superfine) sugar
- ½ tsp sesame oil

It couldn't be easier to transform this humble selection of veg into yet another gluten-free game-changer. Imagine veg that melts in your mouth, coated in a light, crispy and crunchy batter... then make it a reality! The dip really makes this one, so it's definitely worth throwing together and only takes a minute to make.

Pour the vegetable oil into a large, heavy-based saucepan, making sure it is no more than half full. Place over a medium heat and heat for about 15 minutes until it reaches 170°C / 340°F – test the temperature with a cooking thermometer or by using the wooden spoon handle test (page 19).

While the oil is heating, prepare your veg. Chop your red pepper into 1cm / ½in strips and your courgette and aubergine into 1cm / ½in thick discs. Slice your sweet potato into 5mm / ¼in thick discs (cut the slices in half if they're really big). Try your best to roughly stick to these measurements so everything cooks at the same speed.

Combine all the dry batter ingredients in a large mixing bowl. Mix until consistent, then add your carbonated water and whisk together until smooth and without lumps.

Spread the flour onto a large plate. Take a third of your prepared vegetables and roll them around in the flour until well coated. Once your oil is hot, take a few pieces of your coated veg and dip into the batter, ensuring they are well coated. Carefully lower into the hot oil. It should calmly bubble as they cook, without excessive spitting.

Cook for 2–3 minutes until puffy and golden (sweet potato should take around 7–8 minutes – briefly remove them and stab with a fork to make sure they're all nice and soft in the middle before you remove them for good).

Once cooked, use a slotted spoon to remove the tempura and transfer to a wire rack set over a baking tray to drain.

In a small serving dish, mix together the dipping sauce ingredients and serve immediately.

TIP:
Give the batter a regular mix, as the cornflour will sink to the bottom of the mixture after a few minutes.

BEST EVER 3-INGREDIENT
Yorkshire Puddings

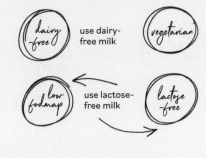

dairy free — use dairy-free milk

vegetarian

low fodmap — use lactose-free milk

lactose free

MAKES · 12

TAKES · 30 MINUTES

- Vegetable oil, for the tray
- 200g / 2 cups cornflour (cornstarch)
- 6 eggs
- 300ml / 1¼ cups milk

My Yorkshire puddings have developed a reputation of their own on the blog, so naturally, they had to be in this book. Everyone loves them because they rise even more than muggle Yorkshire puds and they're super crisp on the outside. Oh and they only need 3 simple ingredients!

Preheat your oven to 200°C fan / 220°C / 425°F.

Grab a muffin tray and add just over 1 teaspoon of oil to each of the holes. Place in the oven for 10-15 minutes until the oil is super hot - basically spitting!

Meanwhile, add your cornflour to a large mixing bowl, crack in your eggs and whisk together. Once thoroughly combined, gradually add the milk, whisking in between additions. Pour the batter into a jug (pitcher) so it's easier to pour.

Next you need to be quick! Remove your muffin tray from the oven and immediately pour batter into each hole until just under three-quarters full. They should sizzle a little as you pour the batter in. Get them back in the oven asap!

Cook for around 15-20 minutes until golden and risen - never open the oven door during their bake as this will ruin them! Once you can see that they're huge and fully risen, give them a little extra time to crisp up as this will reduce the amount they deflate once out of the oven.

Remove from the oven and serve up immediately with a delicious roast dinner and my lazy gluten-free gravy (page 33).

TIP:
You could use tapioca starch instead of cornflour. This recipe also works perfectly for toad in the hole!

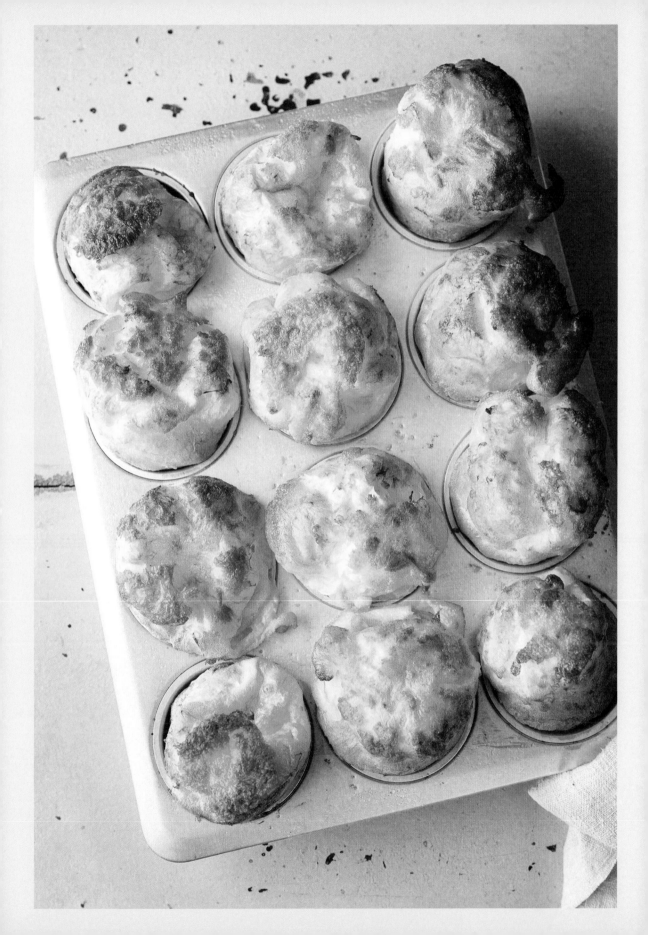

Cheesy Garlic
BREAD PIZZA

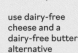

use dairy-free cheese and a dairy-free butter alternative

MAKES · 2

TAKES · 25 MINUTES

- 1 quantity of gluten-free pizza dough (page 47)
- Gluten-free plain (all-purpose) flour, for dusting

For the toppings

- 30g / 2 tbsp butter, melted
- 30ml / 2 tbsp garlic-infused oil
- Handful of fresh parsley, chopped, plus extra (optional) to serve
- Maldon (flaky) sea salt
- 80g / 3oz mozzarella cheese, thinly sliced

I can never get enough of that super thin and crispy base, topped with a quick garlic butter and lots of stringy cheese. It's perfect alongside pasta or as a starter – just make sure you save a slice for me!

Place your pizza dough (having rested it for 30 minutes) on a lightly floured surface.

Cut the dough in half and use a floured rolling pin to roll it out to a 5mm / ⅛in thickness. Aim for a nice, round shape that'll fit into your (large) frying pan – I find it easiest to roll it a little bigger than my frying pan, then cut around the base of the frying pan to ensure it fits perfectly. If the edges are a little cracked, simply use your fingers to gently shape the edges until smooth.

Place the frying pan over a high heat. Once heated, carefully transfer your dough to the dry pan, using a cake lifter or pizza peel. Cook on one side for 2 minutes, then flip and cook on the other side for a further 1 minute, pressing down firmly on the pizza base using a spatula – this encourages the base to puff up a little. Remove from the pan and repeat with the other half of your dough.

Preheat the oven to 200°C fan / 220°C / 425°F.

While the oven is heating, prepare the toppings. In a small bowl, mix your melted butter and garlic-infused oil together, then add the parsley. Generously brush this over the pizza bases, then top with a sprinkling of sea salt. Finally, top with the mozzarella.

Cook in the oven for 8–10 minutes until the cheese is nicely browned and golden. You can either cook them on a pizza tray, or put them straight onto the oven shelf.

Finish with some more chopped parsley, if you like, then slice and serve hot.

TIP:
After you've fried the pizza bases on both sides, they can then be frozen. The next time you fancy cheesy garlic bread pizza, simply top the frozen bases and cook for an extra couple of minutes.

Takeaway-style
EGG-FRIED RICE

 lactose free

 low fodmap — use 45g / ⅓ cup of frozen peas instead

 dairy free

 vegetarian

SERVES · 3

TAKES · 15 MINUTES

- 190g / 1 cup white long-grain rice
- 1 egg
- Pinch of salt
- 3 tbsp vegetable oil
- 4 tbsp sesame oil
- 3 tbsp gluten-free soy sauce (or use gluten-free dark soy sauce, page 35)
- 75g / ⅔ cup frozen peas

This simple side dish is a staple in every Chinese takeaway order, unless you're gluten-free. Fortunately, you can now make it whenever you like! For best results, allow your cooked rice to fully cool, then place in the fridge overnight for the ultimate takeaway-style finish.

Cook your rice according to the packet instructions (steamed works best here) and allow to cool completely, if you have time – ideally pop the rice into an airtight container and chill in the fridge overnight.

Crack the egg into a small bowl, add the salt and briefly beat with a fork.

Add the vegetable oil to a wok and place over a medium heat. Once hot, add the beaten egg and allow to sit for around 30 seconds, then stir to break up the egg into chunks. Add in your cooked rice and stir to break it up. Once it's a little more separated, add in your sesame oil and stir well to coat all of the rice and egg.

Add your soy sauce and stir again so the rice is nicely coated and doesn't look so white.

Stir in your frozen peas and stir-fry for 5 minutes or until the rice starts to look a little crispy in places. If you didn't have time to allow your rice to fully cool or chill in the fridge, you'll likely need to fry for a little longer to reach that point.

Making it vegan?
Omit the egg and use crumbled firm tofu, mixed with a pinch of ground turmeric for colour.

STEAK
Bake

use a low FODMAP stock cube and ensure browning is onion/garlic-free

MAKES · 4

TAKES · 40 MINUTES

- 1 quantity of gluten-free rough puff pastry (page 28)
- 1 egg, beaten

For the filling

- 250g / 9oz beef sirloin (short loin) steak
- 1 tbsp vegetable oil
- 1 tbsp gluten-free plain (all-purpose) flour
- 200ml / generous ¾ cup gluten-free beef stock
- ¼ tsp gravy browning sauce
- ¼ tsp black pepper

When I asked you guys what you'd eat if you could suddenly eat gluten again for one day, so many of you said the same thing: steak bake! With golden, puffy layers of buttery pastry, packed with tender, juicy beef, I can definitely understand why. So this one is for all you guys who miss this!

Firstly, make your filling. Using a sharp knife, chop your sirloin steak into small chunks that are around 2 x 1cm / ¾ x ½in.

Add the vegetable oil to a large pan and place over a medium heat. Add your chopped beef and fry until lightly browned on all sides. Stir in your flour until all the beef is evenly coated. Pour in your stock, gravy browning sauce and black pepper. Bring to the boil and simmer until the mixture reduces to form a nice, thick gravy. Turn off the heat and allow to cool briefly.

Preheat your oven to 200°C fan / 220°C / 425°F and line a large baking tray with non-stick baking parchment.

Place the pastry on a large sheet of non-stick baking parchment. Cut it in half, rewrap one portion in cling film (plastic wrap) and place in the fridge while you roll out the first pastry portion into a large rectangle, around 20 x 30cm / 8 x 12in, and 2mm / ¹⁄₁₆in thick. Cut the rectangle into 4 smaller rectangles, each 15 x 10cm / 6 x 4in (you need 2 rectangles per steak bake). Brush the edges of one of the rectangles with a little beaten egg.

Spoon a good tablespoon of steak filling into the centre of two of your rectangles, then place your remaining rectangles of pastry on top, pressing down around all the edges. Use a fork to seal the edges. Score 4–6 lines diagonally across the top of each bake with a sharp knife and then brush the top with beaten egg. Transfer your steak bakes to your lined baking tray.

Repeat, using the rest of your pastry and filling. Cook in the oven for 20 minutes until golden, then remove from the oven and enjoy served warm.

TIPS:

Remember that when using rough puff pastry, you cannot simply just reroll it (or any off-cuts) into a ball. You'll destroy the layers you've spent time creating! If you do have any off-cuts, you can always bake them and roll them in cinnamon sugar for a sweet, buttery treat. If you don't have time to make your own pastry, use store-bought gluten-free pastry instead.

Making it veggie?
Simply use the filling from my veggie samosas over on page 85 in place of the steak filling, to make a spicy veggie bake.

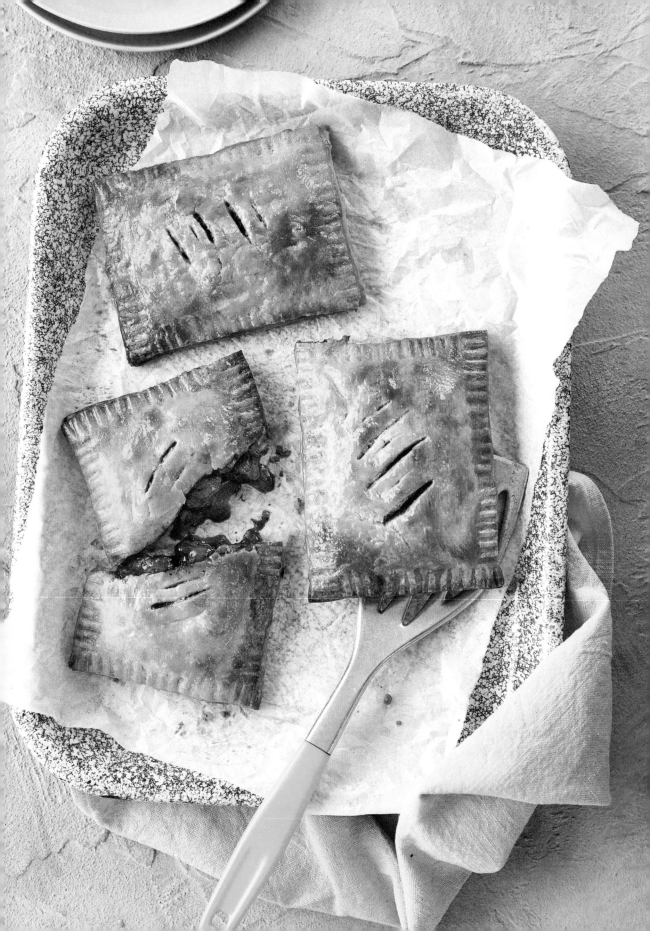

5-Ingredient SCOTCH EGGS

ensure the breadcrumbs are low FODMAP

MAKES · 4

TAKES · 45 MINUTES

- 5 medium eggs
- 500g / 18oz pork mince (ground pork)
- 3 tsp dried sage
- 50g / 6 tbsp gluten-free plain (all-purpose) flour
- 60g / 1 cup gluten-free breadcrumbs (page 32 or store-bought)
- Vegetable oil, for cooking
- Salt and white pepper

With a perfectly cooked, soft-boiled egg encased in tender, lightly seasoned sausage meat and crispy breadcrumbs, Scotch eggs are the perfect all-in-one snack. The addition of white pepper is my secret ingredient as it adds a subtle peppery heat, but of course it's entirely optional if you don't have any to hand.

Add 4 of your eggs (shell on) to a large saucepan, cover in cold water and bring to the boil. Make sure you don't cook the fifth egg as we'll need it later! Turn down the heat and gently simmer for 4 minutes, then immediately remove the eggs and place straight into a bowl of cold water – the colder, the better!

While your eggs are cooling, grab a large mixing bowl and add your pork mince and sage. Season with a little salt and 1 teaspoon of white pepper. Give it a good mix so it's all nicely dispersed. Divide the mixture into four equal pieces and shape each piece into a ball.

Grab two plates and a small bowl. Crack your last egg into the bowl and briefly beat with a fork. Add your flour to one plate and spread out, then add your breadcrumbs to the other plate and spread out once again.

Carefully peel your cooled eggs and make sure there's no shell lurking about!

First of all, grab one of your pork balls and place on a large sheet of cling film (plastic wrap). Fold the cling film over it and, using your hands, flatten the ball into a rough square about 5mm / ¼in thick. Peel back the cling film.

Take one of your boiled eggs and roll it around gently on the flour plate to coat, then place on your flattened pork square. Using the cling film, wrap the mince around the egg until it's completely covered, making sure you can't see the egg at all. Remove the cling film and set aside ready to shape the next one.

Roll the pork-covered egg on the flour plate until nicely dusted on all sides, then place the ball in the beaten egg bowl and gently roll around until well coated with egg. Finally, roll on the breadcrumb plate until totally covered. Set aside and repeat for the remaining boiled eggs.

You've got two options on how to finish your Scotch eggs: frying them, or baking them in the oven. The oven is fine, but frying gives them a miles better finish and a softer middle.

To fry, pour enough vegetable oil into a large, heavy-based pan to fill it by a third. Place over a medium heat for 10 minutes until heated to 170°C / 340°F – test the temperature with a cooking thermometer or by using the wooden spoon handle test (page 19).

Gently lower 2 of the Scotch eggs into the hot oil and cook for 8 minutes, turning halfway through. Ensure the oil doesn't get too hot or they will brown before the pork gets a chance to cook right through. Once cooked, remove from the oil using a slotted spoon and place onto a wire rack set over a baking tray to drain while you fry the remaining Scotch eggs.

To cook in the oven, preheat your oven to 200°C fan / 220°C / 425°F. Place your Scotch eggs on a lightly greased baking tray (or spray with a little vegetable oil). Cook in the oven for 25 minutes, turning them over halfway through. They won't brown as much as if frying them, but they'll taste almost identical.

Pictured on page 99

Making it veggie?
Use 'meaty' vegetarian sausages instead of pork, and remove all of the filling from the sausage casing.

PROPER
Pork Pies

use lard instead of butter for greasing

MAKES · 12

TAKES · 1 HOUR

- Butter or lard, for greasing
- 1 quantity of gluten-free hot water crust pastry (page 29)
- Gluten-free plain (all-purpose) flour, for dusting
- 1 egg, beaten

For the filling

- 500g / 18oz pork mince (ground pork)
- 100g / 3½oz smoked streaky bacon, diced
- 3 tsp dried sage
- 1 tsp ground nutmeg (optional)
- ½ tsp salt
- ½ tsp black pepper

These mini savoury pies are encased in golden, buttery pastry and filled with a meaty pork filling. Enjoy them cold for lunch, warmed up for dinner with relish, or as a game-changing 'I can't believe I can even eat this' snack.

Add all the filling ingredients to a large mixing bowl and mix thoroughly, then cover and keep chilled until needed.

Grab a muffin tray and, using kitchen paper, lightly grease all of the holes with butter or lard. Remove your hot water crust pastry from the fridge and preheat your oven to 200°C fan / 220°C / 425°F.

Generously flour your work surface and rolling pin. Place your dough on the work surface and knead for 1 minute, adding more flour as necessary. Cut off one third of the dough and put it to one side, covering it with a tea (dish) towel to stop it drying out.

Roll the remaining dough out to a large rectangle about 3mm / ⅛in thick, ensuring your surface and rolling pin remain well floured so it doesn't stick. Use a 10cm / 4in round biscuit (cookie) cutter to cut out as many circles as you can from the dough. You may have to reroll the off-cuts once more to get as many as 12.

Using a palette knife, lift the round shapes into the holes of your greased muffin tray. Gently push the pastry in, using your fingers, ensuring there's a 3mm / ⅛in overhang by encouraging the pastry over the edge of your muffin hole. Repeat until you've used up your pastry.

Re-flour your work surface and roll out the reserved piece of dough to a 3mm / ⅛in thickness. Use an 8cm / 3in plain pastry cutter to cut out 12 circles for the lids.

Next, add the pork filling to your pastry cases, filling them to just slightly below the top of the pastry. Brush the edges of the pastry with a little beaten egg. Use a palette knife to transfer the pastry lids to the tops of the pastry cases. Crimp the edges together using a fork, taking care not to disturb the other pies.

Brush each pie with beaten egg. Lastly, make a small hole in the very centre of the top of each lid by gently prodding with a sharp knife and twisting. Bake in the oven for 20 minutes, then reduce the oven temperature to 160°C fan / 180°C / 350°F and bake for another 15 minutes, until golden.

Serve with a little relish on the side and enjoy hot or cold.

Pictured on page 99

ULTIMATE
Sausage Rolls

low lactose

low fodmap

dairy free

MAKES · 12

TAKES · 45 MINUTES

- 1 quantity of gluten-free rough puff pastry (page 28)
- 5 tbsp wholegrain mustard
- 1 egg, beaten
- Handful of sesame seeds

For the filling

- 500g / 18oz pork mince (ground pork)
- 3 tsp dried sage
- 1 tsp white pepper
- Salt

If you've missed mini sausage rolls wrapped in buttery, puffy, flaky pastry as much as I have, then you'll have no qualms about making them yourself! Enjoy as a snack, or whip them up whenever you need some party food canapés.

Preheat your oven to 180°C fan / 200°C / 400°F.

In a large mixing bowl, add your pork mince, sage, pepper and a generous pinch of salt. Give it a good mix so it's all nicely dispersed and mash with a fork until the mince is as broken down as possible.

Place the pastry on a large sheet of non-stick baking parchment. Cut the pastry in half, rewrap one portion in cling film (plastic wrap) and place in the fridge while you roll out the first portion into a large rectangle, around 20 x 30cm / 8 x 12in, and 3mm / ⅛in thick. With a shorter side closest to you, spread half your mustard 1cm / ½in off-centre in a 2.5cm / 1in line from top to bottom.

Next, spoon half of your pork mixture on top of the long line of mustard from top to bottom. It should be just under 2.5cm / 1in high. Brush the smaller side of the pastry with a little beaten egg. Fold the larger side of the pastry over the filling. Using your fingers, gently form the pastry around the filling to remove any gaps.

Trim the excess pastry alongside the filling, leaving just 1cm / ½in of pastry along the seam. Crimp the pastry all along the seam, using a fork, to securely seal it shut.

Brush the sausage roll with beaten egg and use a sharp knife to cut diagonal slashes in the top of the pastry, then sprinkle half your sesame seeds all over the top. Repeat with the other half of your pastry, filling and seeds so that you have two long sausage rolls.

Using the baking parchment to lift them, transfer your sausage rolls to separate baking trays. Cook for 30–35 minutes until golden, then remove from the oven and place onto a wire rack to cool (you can serve them hot or cold).

Slice each long sausage roll into 6 smaller sausage rolls and serve with a little relish on the side.

TIPS:
Remember that when using rough puff pastry, you cannot simply just reroll it (or any off-cuts) into a ball. You'll destroy the layers you've spent time creating! If you do have any off-cuts, you can always bake them and roll them in cinnamon sugar for a sweet, buttery treat.

If you don't have time to make your own pastry, use store-bought gluten-free pastry instead.

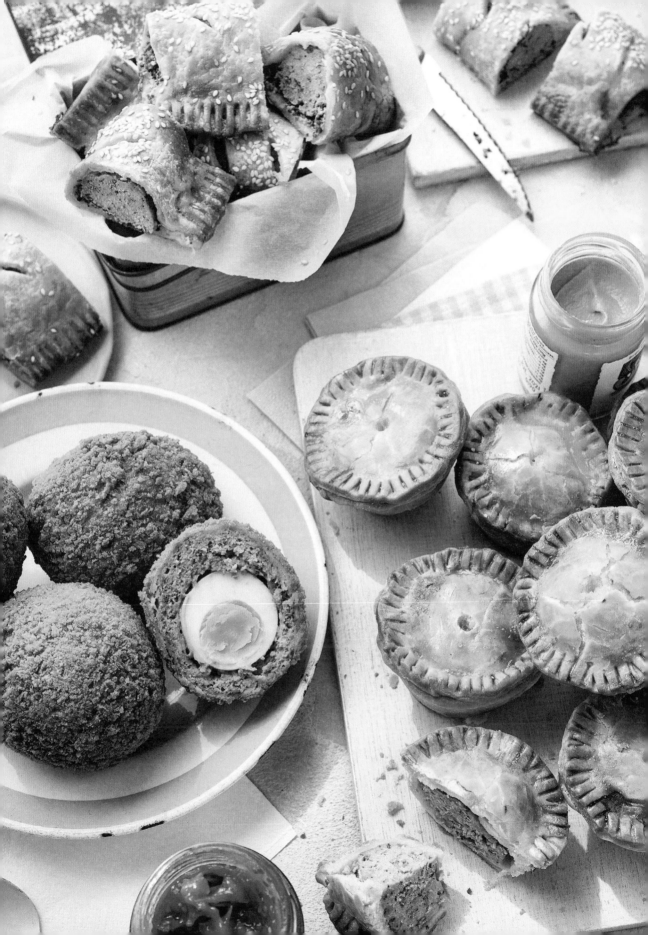

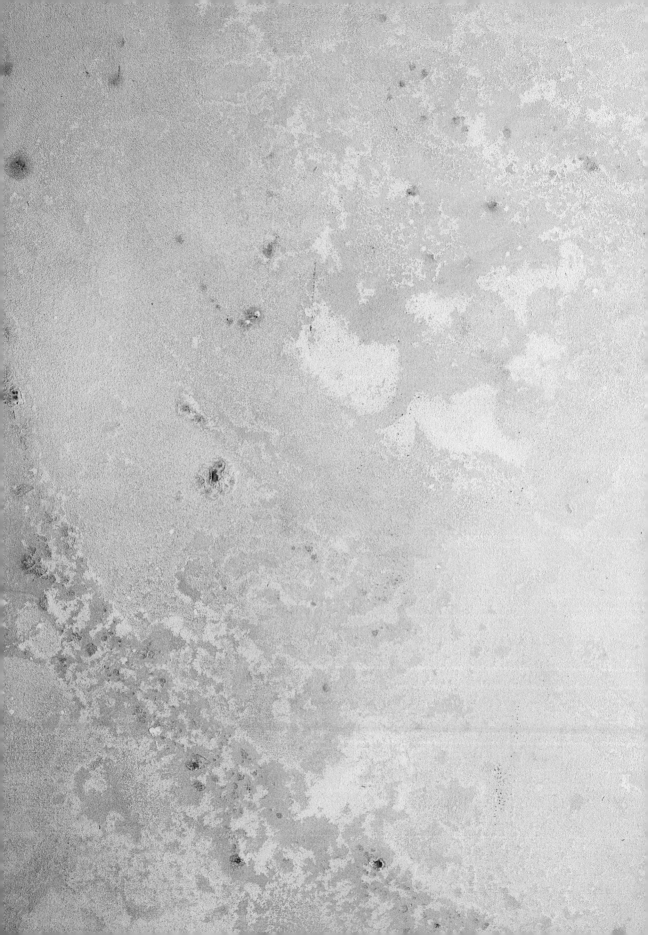

Fakeaways

Takeaways often mean food prepared in a very small kitchen where there's gluten *everywhere*. Of course, making it at home negates the nightmare of cross-contamination. Then, removing or replacing the gluten-containing ingredients makes it edible – hooray!

But there's still one crucial factor here: does it still taste *exactly* like the food you'd get from the takeaway? Because if it doesn't... then it's not really a proper 'fakeaway' is it?

That's why, with my boyfriend Mark's help, I set out to recreate all of my takeaway favourites, without gluten and without compromise. Not only would you never know they're gluten-free, but nobody would ever know these weren't made by a real takeaway either.

So welcome to my ultimate gluten-free takeaway – may I take your order?

Sweet and Sour
CRISPY CHICKEN, PORK OR PRAWN BALLS

use water instead of milk

use lactose-free milk

SERVES · 4

TAKES · 40 MINUTES

- 1.5l / 6½ cups vegetable oil
- 50g / 6 tbsp gluten-free plain (all-purpose) flour
- 400g / 14oz chicken breast fillets, chopped into 2.5cm / 1in cubes **OR** 400g / 14oz pork tenderloin, chopped into 2.5cm / 1in cubes **OR** 350g / 12¼oz shelled and deveined raw prawns (shrimp)

For the batter

- 200g / 1½ cups gluten-free plain (all-purpose) flour
- 1 tsp gluten-free baking powder
- ½ tsp salt
- 200ml / generous ¾ cup milk or water

For the sauce

- 175ml / ¾ cup pineapple juice (or smooth orange juice)
- 70ml / generous ¼ cup white rice vinegar
- 20g / 1½ tbsp light brown sugar
- 175g / ¾ cup tomato ketchup
- 3 tbsp cornflour (cornstarch)
- 6 tbsp cold water

Yep, these are exactly like the big, chunky chicken, pork or prawn balls that you'd see on the menu at your local Chinese takeaway. The batter is thick, golden and super crispy – perfect drenched in my quick, takeaway-style sweet and sour sauce.

For the sauce, add all the ingredients except the cornflour and water to a large saucepan and place over a medium heat. Bring to the boil, stirring occasionally, then reduce to a simmer. Mix the cornflour with the water and add to the pan, stirring it in immediately until it disappears. Simmer until the sauce thickens, then take off the heat and place to one side.

Next, add the vegetable oil to a deep, heavy-based saucepan and place over a medium heat. Heat for around 15 minutes, until it reaches 170°C / 340°F; test the temperature with a cooking thermometer, or by using the wooden spoon handle test (page 19).

While your oil is heating, combine the ingredients for the batter in a large mixing bowl and whisk together until smooth, thick and consistent. Allow to rest for 5 minutes.

Meanwhile, spread the 50g / 6 tbsp of flour out on a large plate. Add your cubed chicken, pork or raw prawns in batches to the plate and toss until they're all evenly coated in flour. Transfer to the batter, briefly mix until fully submerged and nicely coated.

Once your oil is hot enough, carefully lower the batter-coated pieces of chicken/pork/prawn into the oil, 5 or 6 at a time. Lower them in slightly apart to prevent sticking. They should sizzle nicely as you place them in.

Cook for 10 minutes if using chicken or pork, or 5–7 minutes if using prawns. Once cooked, remove from the oil using a slotted spoon and place onto a wire rack suspended over a baking tray to drain.

Reheat your sauce briefly, if needed. Serve up with my egg-fried rice (page 93) and don't forget to make some prawn toast (page 80) to serve alongside too.

Pictured on page 104

Making it vegan? Or veggie?
Use a block of extra-firm tofu in place of the chicken, pork or prawns, cut into 2.5cm / 1in chunks, and proceed with the recipe as directed. If vegan, use water instead of milk.

SALT & PEPPER SHREDDED
Chilli Chicken

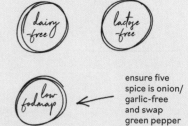

ensure five spice is onion/garlic-free and swap green pepper for red

SERVES · 2

TAKES · 40 MINUTES

- 250g / 9oz chicken breast fillets, thinly sliced
- 500ml / 2 cups vegetable oil
- 2 tbsp garlic-infused oil
- 1 green (bell) pepper, chopped
- 1 carrot, thinly sliced on the diagonal
- ¼ tsp dried chilli flakes (optional)
- Handful of spring onion (scallion) greens, chopped

For the seasoning

- ½ tsp Chinese five spice
- ½ tsp ground ginger
- ½ tsp black pepper
- ½ tsp salt

For the coating

- 90g / scant 1 cup cornflour (cornstarch)
- 135g / 1 cup gluten-free plain (all-purpose) flour
- 1 tsp gluten-free baking powder
- ¼ tsp salt
- 2 eggs

Here's yet another Chinese takeaway classic that I could otherwise only dream of eating! Light and crispy chicken generously sprinkled with a mildly spicy, salt and pepper seasoning.

In a small bowl, combine all the ingredients for the seasoning and place to one side. (You can make a big batch of this and store it in an airtight container for future meals.)

Mix all the dry ingredients for the coating together in a large bowl. Crack the eggs into a medium-sized bowl and beat with a fork.

Add a third of your chicken slices to the dry ingredients bowl and toss until evenly coated, then transfer them to the beaten egg bowl and toss once again until well coated. Finally, transfer them back to the dry ingredients bowl and toss until totally covered, occasionally squeezing the chicken so that the flour compacts onto it as much as possible. Repeat with the remaining chicken, in 2 more batches.

Grab a sturdy wok and pour in the vegetable oil so it is about 2cm / ¾in deep. Place over a medium heat for 8-10 minutes or until it reaches 170°C / 340°F - test with a cooking thermometer or by using the wooden spoon handle test (page 19). In 2 batches, lower the coated chicken strips into the oil - they should sizzle as you place them in.

Cook for around 3 minutes on each side or until the batter is golden and crispy, then remove with a slotted spoon and transfer to a wire rack placed over a baking tray to drain. Once they're all done, refry all of them in the oil for another 3-4 minutes, in 2 batches.

This will make them super crunchy! Place them back onto the wire rack to drain once more.

Heat your garlic-infused oil in a large frying pan over a medium heat. Add in your green pepper and carrot and stir-fry for 3-4 minutes until slightly browned. Add your cooked chicken and stir for a minute or so. Sprinkle in a third of your seasoning (tipping it all in at once won't give you even coverage), give it a good stir and repeat until all of your seasoning is used.

Take off the heat and add the dried chilli flakes if you'd like a little extra kick. Throw your spring onion greens into the pan and mix once more before serving with my egg-fried rice (page 93).

TIP:
You can also use this seasoning blend on cooked oven chips to make your own salt and pepper chips just like you'd get from the takeaway.

Pictured on page 104

Making it veggie?
Use a block of extra-firm tofu cut into 2.5cm / 1in chunks in place of the chicken, and proceed with the recipe as directed.

Making it vegan?
Use tofu as described above and instead of using an egg to coat the tofu, mix 100ml / generous ⅓ cup soy milk with 2 tsp lemon juice. Allow to rest for 10 minutes before using.

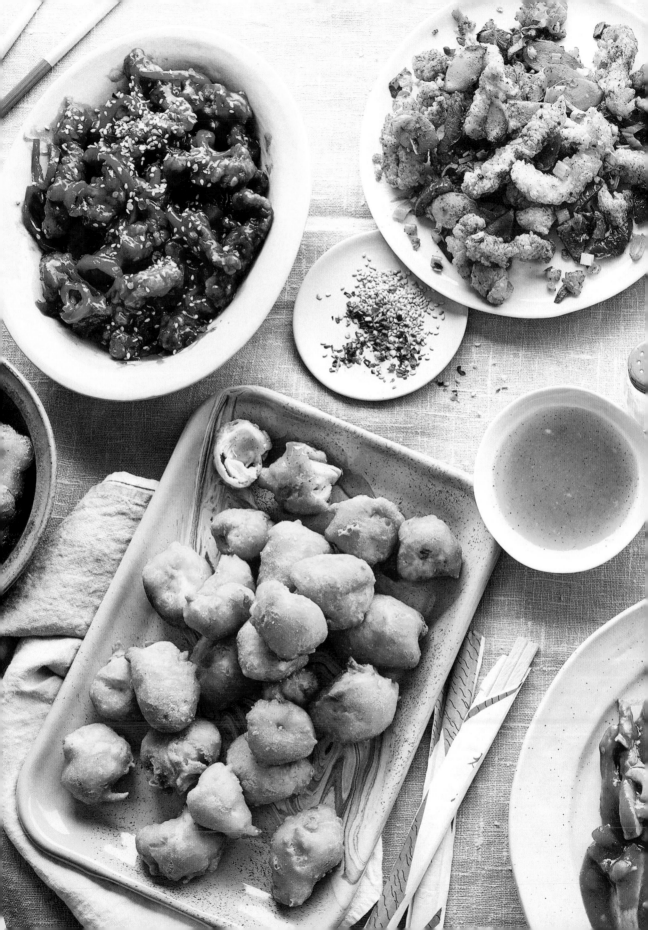

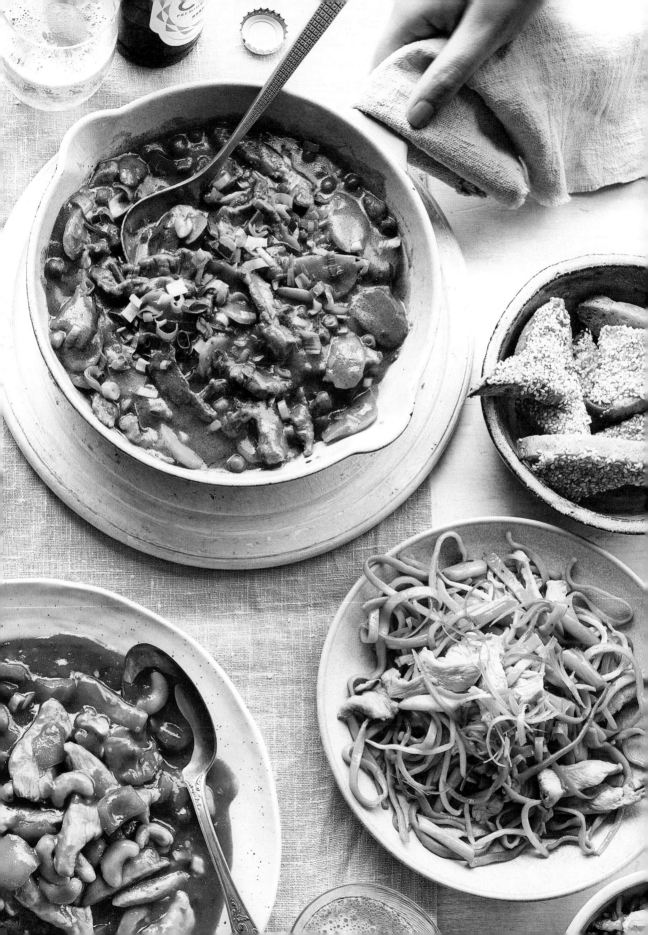

Quick
KUNG PAO CHICKEN

SERVES · 2

TAKES · 15 MINUTES

- 1 tbsp garlic-infused oil
- 250g / 9oz chicken breast fillets, thinly sliced
- 1 green (bell) pepper, chopped
- 1 tbsp gluten-free plain (all-purpose) flour
- Handful of cashew nuts
- Handful of spring onion (scallion) greens, chopped

For the sauce

- 100g / scant ½ cup tomato ketchup
- 1 tbsp gluten-free soy sauce (or use gluten-free dark soy sauce, page 35)
- 80g / 6 tbsp light brown sugar
- 1 tbsp minced ginger paste (optional)
- 2 tbsp white rice vinegar
- 230ml / scant 1 cup water
- 2 tsp miso paste (ensure gluten-free)
- 1 tsp dried chilli flakes or Sichuan pepper
- 1 tsp balsamic vinegar

I can't describe how much I've missed eating this, so I'll describe what it tastes like instead! Think tender chicken and chunky cashew nuts in a mildly spicy sauce, brimming with that unmistakable, deep, sweet and savoury Kung Pao flavour. For a little more spice, sprinkle an extra ½ teaspoon of dried chilli flakes on top before serving.

Combine all the ingredients for the sauce in a small mixing bowl, giving it a good mix until everything is well combined.

Heat up your garlic-infused oil in a wok over a medium-high heat and fry your sliced chicken for 1 minute. Add in the green pepper and stir-fry for another 2–3 minutes, then add in your flour. Mix immediately so that the chicken and pepper are evenly coated in the flour.

Add in your sauce and give it a good stir until all the lumps of flour are gone. Bring to the boil and simmer for 5 minutes or until the sauce begins to thicken. Throw in the cashew nuts and chopped spring onion greens, then mix.

Serve up with my egg-fried (page 93).

Pictured on page 105

Making it veggie? Or vegan? Use a block of extra-firm tofu cut into 2.5cm / 1in chunks, coated in cornflour (cornstarch), in place of the chicken, and proceed with the recipe as directed.

Chinese Take-Out Curry WITH CHICKEN OR BEEF

SERVES · 2

TAKES · 20 MINUTES

- 1 tbsp garlic-infused oil
- 250g / 9oz chicken breast fillets or beef sirloin (short loin) steak, thinly sliced
- 1 carrot, thinly sliced on the diagonal
- 400ml / 1⅔ cups gluten-free chicken stock
- 1 tsp gluten-free soy sauce
- 40g / 1½oz creamed coconut block (optional)
- 1 tsp maple syrup (optional)
- 30g / 1oz frozen peas
- Handful of spring onion (scallion) greens, chopped

For the spice blend

- 1½ tbsp gluten-free-plain (all-purpose) flour
- 2 tsp mild curry powder
- ½ tsp dried chilli flakes (optional)
- ½ tsp Chinese five spice

So many of you have made my takeaway-style Chinese chicken curry over the years. It's mildly spicy with a lovely, thick curry sauce that goes so well with egg-fried rice. I thought I'd revamp it and make it a little creamier, as well as highlight how it's amazing with beef too – trust me, you'll love it!

In a small bowl, combine all the ingredients for the spice blend. Place to one side. (You can always make a huge batch of this and store it in an airtight container for future meals.)

Place your wok over a medium-high heat and add your garlic-infused oil. Once heated, add the thinly sliced chicken or beef strips. Stir-fry for 2 minutes, then add your carrot. Continue to stir-fry for another 2–3 minutes.

Next, add your spice blend and immediately stir so that it coats all of the carrot and chicken/beef strips. Once everything is nicely coated, add your stock and soy sauce, immediately followed by your creamed coconut and maple syrup, if using. Then add your frozen peas.

Bring to the boil and simmer for around 10 minutes or until the sauce becomes lovely and thick. Throw in your spring onion greens and mix once more before serving up with my egg-fried rice (page 93).

Pictured on page 105

Making it veggie? Or vegan?
Use a 400g / 14oz can of chickpeas (garbanzo beans) instead of beef or chicken – add these once the sauce has reduced. Use a gluten-free vegetable/vegan stock cube and proceed with the recipe as directed.

Making it low FODMAP?
Use a low FODMAP stock cube, skip the creamed coconut and ensure the five spice and curry powder are onion/garlic-free.

Crispy Chilli
BEEF

SERVES · 2

TAKES · 45 MINUTES

- 250g / 9oz beef sirloin (short loin) steak
- 500ml / 2 cups vegetable oil
- 1 tbsp garlic-infused oil
- 1 red (bell) pepper, chopped into thin strips
- 1 tbsp gluten-free plain (all-purpose) flour
- 2 tbsp sesame seeds (optional)

For the coating

- 90g / scant 1 cup cornflour (cornstarch)
- 135g / 1 cup gluten-free plain (all-purpose) flour
- 1 tsp gluten-free baking powder
- ¼ tsp salt
- 2 eggs

For the sauce

- 100g / scant ½ cup tomato ketchup
- 3 tbsp gluten-free soy sauce (or use gluten-free dark soy sauce, page 35)
- 80g / 6 tbsp light brown sugar
- 1 tbsp minced ginger paste (optional)
- 2 tbsp rice wine vinegar
- 230ml / scant 1 cup water
- 2 tbsp gluten-free brown sauce
- 2 tsp gluten-free Worcestershire sauce (optional)
- 1 tsp dried chilli flakes

I honestly thought I'd never eat this ever again after having to go gluten-free. And yep, those super crispy, crunchy strips of beef in a sticky, mildly spicy sauce are now back on the menu. For a little more spice, sprinkle an extra ½ teaspoon of dried chilli flakes on top before serving.

To prepare your beef, place the steak between two sheets of cling film (plastic wrap) and bash until flat, using a rolling pin or meat mallet. Thinly slice into super thin strips – the thinner the better!

Mix all the dry ingredients for the coating together in a large bowl, stirring until evenly combined. Crack the eggs into another bowl and beat with a fork.

Add a third of your beef strips to the dry ingredients and toss until evenly coated. Transfer to the beaten egg bowl and toss until well coated, then transfer them back to the dry ingredients and toss until totally covered, occasionally squeezing the beef so that the flour compacts onto it as much as possible. Repeat with the remaining beef, in 2 batches.

Grab a sturdy wok and pour in the vegetable oil so it is about 2cm / ¾in deep. Place over a medium heat for 8–10 minutes or until it reaches 170°C / 340°F – test with a cooking thermometer, or by using the wooden spoon handle test (page 19). In 2 batches, carefully lower your coated beef strips into the oil – they should sizzle nicely as you place them in. Cook for around 4–5 minutes until

the batter is golden and crispy, then remove from the oil with a slotted spoon and place onto a wire rack set over a baking tray, to drain.

Once they're done, refry all of your beef in the oil for another 3–4 minutes, again in 2 batches. This is the key to making them super crunchy, so don't skip this part. Place them back onto the wire rack to drain once more while you prepare the sauce.

Combine all the sauce ingredients in a small bowl; place to one side while you heat up your garlic-infused oil in a large frying pan over a medium-high heat. Once heated, add in your red pepper and stir-fry for 2–3 minutes. Add in the 1 tablespoon of flour, mixing it in immediately so that the pepper is evenly coated in the flour.

Once coated, add in your sauce, give it a good stir until all visible lumps of flour are gone. Bring to the boil and simmer for 5 minutes or until the sauce begins to thicken. Add your crispy beef strips and stir until totally covered. Top with the sesame seeds and a sprinkling of dried chilli flakes and serve immediately.

Pictured on page 104

Making it veggie? Or vegan?
Use a block of extra-firm tofu cut into 2.5cm / 1in chunks in place of the beef, and proceed with the recipe as directed. If making it vegan, instead of using an egg to coat the tofu, mix 100ml / generous ⅓ cup soy milk with 2 tsp lemon juice. Allow to rest for 10 minutes before using. Omit Worcestershire sauce.

Chow mein
WITH CHICKEN OR BEEF

SERVES · 2

TAKES · 15 MINUTES

- 2 tbsp garlic-infused oil
- 250g / 9oz chicken breast fillets or beef sirloin (short loin) steak, thinly sliced
- 1 carrot, thinly sliced on the diagonal
- 250g / 9oz gluten-free egg noodles (page 34, or see recipe intro for store-bought 'cheat')
- 4 tbsp gluten-free soy sauce (or use gluten-free dark soy sauce, page 35)
- 2 tsp sesame oil
- Pinch of caster (superfine) sugar
- Handful of beansprouts
- 2 handfuls of spring onion (scallion) greens, chopped, plus extra to serve

This one is a real game-changer! Either make your own gluten-free egg noodles (page 34) for the 'real deal' experience, or cheat using store-bought gluten-free spaghetti that's been cooked and left out to dry for a couple of hours. Allowing it to air-dry gives it the chewier bite of egg noodles. Feel free to make spring rolls (page 81) to serve alongside your chow mein.

Add your garlic-infused oil to a wok and place over a medium heat. Once heated, stir-fry the chicken or beef strips for 1 minute before adding the carrot. Continue to stir-fry for 2 minutes until the carrot softens.

Add your noodles, soy sauce, sesame oil and sugar. Stir-fry until everything is well coated, then add the beansprouts and spring onion greens.

Mix in, turn up the heat to high and stir-fry for 2 minutes. Remove from the heat, garnish with a few more spring onion greens and serve up.

Pictured on page 105

Making it veggie?
Replace the chicken with half a red pepper, cut into strips, and two handfuls of chopped mushrooms.

Making it vegan?
Follow the advice above to make it veggie and use store-bought gluten-free spaghetti (ensure vegan) instead of my homemade egg noodles.

Quick Beef
IN BLACK BEAN SAUCE

use a low FODMAP stock cube and swap green pepper for more red

SERVES · 2

TAKES · 15 MINUTES

- 2 tbsp canned black beans, drained
- 3 tbsp garlic-infused oil
- 250g / 9oz beef sirloin (short loin) steak, thinly sliced
- ½ green (bell) pepper, chopped
- ½ red (bell) pepper, chopped
- 250ml / 1 cup gluten-free beef stock
- 2 tbsp gluten-free soy sauce (or use gluten-free dark soy sauce, page 35)
- 1 tsp white rice vinegar
- 1 tsp maple syrup
- 1 tbsp cornflour (cornstarch)
- 2 tbsp cold water

I went an entire decade without eating this... but it was well worth the wait! After one bite of tender beef, drenched in that mouth-watering, gravy-like black bean sauce, you'll never want to go without eating it ever again.

Put the black beans into a small bowl. Using a fork, mash them up and add 1 tablespoon of the garlic-infused oil. Mix until well combined and set aside. I usually freeze the rest of my black beans so I can break off a few (and defrost) for the next time that I make this.

Grab a wok, add your remaining oil and place over a high heat.

Add your beef and stir-fry for around 1 minute. Once the beef has browned slightly, add your chopped peppers. Continue to stir-fry for 2–3 minutes until the peppers begin to brown slightly. Add your black bean mixture and turn the heat down to medium. Continue to stir-fry for a minute until the beef and peppers are nicely coated.

Add in your stock, soy sauce, vinegar and maple syrup, bring to the boil then simmer for 3 minutes. Mix the cornflour and cold water together in a small dish, then drizzle this into the wok and immediately stir in.

Serve with egg-fried rice (page 93) and my sticky Chinese-style spare ribs (page 82).

TIP:
You can also make this using chicken breast instead of beef.

Making it veggie? Or vegan?
Replace the beef with baby corn and a thinly sliced carrot. Use a gluten-free vegetable/vegan stock cube and proceed with the recipe as directed.

CRISPY DUCK PANCAKES

with Hoisin Sauce

ensure five spice/miso paste is onion/garlic-free

SERVES · 2–3

TAKES · 1 HOUR 45 MINUTES

- 450g / 1lb duck legs (bone in, skin on)
- 3 tsp Chinese five spice

For the hoisin sauce

- 1 tbsp garlic-infused oil
- 2 tbsp canned black beans, drained
- 2½ tbsp dark brown muscovado sugar
- 1 tsp rice wine vinegar
- 1 tsp sesame oil
- ½ tsp Chinese five spice
- ½ tsp miso paste (ensure gluten-free)
- 250ml / 1 cup water
- 2 tbsp gluten-free soy sauce
- 1 tsp minced ginger paste
- 1 tbsp cornflour (cornstarch)
- 2 tbsp cold water

To serve

- 15 rice paper spring roll wrappers
- 5 spring onion (scallion) greens, cut into thin matchsticks
- ½ cucumber, cut into thin matchsticks

This is a really quick and easy way to prepare crispy duck. I'm tired of only being able to eat these with lettuce wraps, so instead I serve them up with rice paper wrappers. And who could forget my homemade gluten-free hoisin sauce too?

Preheat the oven to 160°C fan / 180°C / 350°F.

Rub the duck legs all over with your five spice, massaging it all in until the legs are all completely and evenly covered. Place the duck in a roasting dish lined with foil and cook in the oven for 1 hour 30 minutes.

Meanwhile, for the hoisin sauce, add all the ingredients except the cornflour and water to a large saucepan and place over a low heat. Bring to the boil and simmer for 5–10 minutes. Mix the cornflour and water in a small dish, drizzle into the wok and immediately stir it in. Once the sauce has thickened, pour it into a small bowl.

Remove the duck from the oven; the skin should be super crispy. Place onto a wire rack set over a baking tray and allow to rest for 10 minutes, then transfer to a plate and, using two forks, shred all of the meat and tear up the crispy skin as best you can.

To construct your duck pancakes, take a rice paper wrapper and dip it in cold water for 5 seconds, immersing it completely. Then place the wrapper on a wooden surface or a damp cloth. After around 10–15 seconds, it should no longer feel plasticky and hard – it should feel more flexible and slightly sticky. Fill with duck, hoisin sauce, spring onion and cucumber. Fold the bottom so that it overlaps the filling, then fold over the sides. Repeat until you've used up all of your duck, keeping each pancake slightly apart so they don't stick together.

Making it vegan? Or veggie?
Instead of using duck, shred 200g / 7oz king oyster mushrooms with two forks. Coat in 3 tsp Chinese five spice, drizzle with 3 tbsp garlic-infused oil, place on a baking tray and roast in the oven at 160°C fan / 180°C / 350°F for 20 minutes.

CHICKEN AND PRAWN
Pad Thai

use no more than 1 tbsp of tamarind paste →

SERVES · 2

TAKES · 20 MINUTES

- 200g / 7oz dried ribbon rice noodles
- 3–4 tbsp vegetable oil
- 150g / 5¼oz chicken breast fillets, thinly sliced
- 175g / 6½oz shelled and deveined raw prawns (shrimp)
- 2 eggs
- Handful of spring onion (scallion) greens
- Handful of beansprouts
- 2 tbsp crushed roasted peanuts (ensure gluten-free)

For the sauce

- 2 tbsp tamarind paste
- 3 tbsp palm sugar or light brown sugar
- 3 tbsp fish sauce
- 2 tbsp garlic-infused oil
- 1 tbsp gluten-free soy sauce
- 3 tbsp water

To serve (optional)

- 1 lime, cut into wedges
- ½ tsp dried chilli flakes

I can't express how much I've missed eating a good pad Thai. Who'd have guessed it was so incredibly simple to make gluten-free? It's packed with tons of sweet, sour and savoury flavours and you can whip it up in 20 minutes.

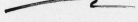

In a small bowl, combine all the sauce ingredients. Prepare your rice noodles according to the packet instructions, drain and set aside.

Heat the oil in a wok over a medium-high heat. Add your chicken and fry until almost sealed, then add your prawns and stir-fry until they begin to colour on both sides.

Move the chicken and prawns to one side of the wok, crack both eggs into the other side of the wok and beat until thoroughly mixed. Keep stirring until it forms nicely scrambled egg chunks. Add in your prepared rice noodles and stir-fry briefly. Add your sauce and toss the noodles until everything is well coated.

Lastly, add in your spring onion greens and beansprouts. Stir-fry once more until the beansprouts begin to soften slightly. Serve with the crushed peanuts on top and, if you fancy, a wedge of lime and the dried chilli flakes.

TIP:
I find that rice noodles that also have a little tapioca starch in them are the best, as they don't break as easily.

Making this veggie? Or vegan?
Use a vegan alternative to fish sauce (available online). Replace the chicken and prawns with a block of extra-firm tofu, cut into 2.5cm / 1in chunks coated in cornflour (cornstarch). If vegan, add 100g / 3½oz of shredded carrot when the recipe calls for eggs.

Chicken
KATSU CURRY

SERVES · 2

TAKES · 40 MINUTES

- 300g / 10½oz chicken breast fillets
- 1 egg
- 50g / 6 tbsp gluten-free plain (all-purpose) flour
- 80g / 1¼ cups gluten-free breadcrumbs (page 32 or store-bought)
- 50ml / 3½ tbsp vegetable oil
- 2 handfuls fresh chives, chopped, to serve

For the katsu sauce

- 2 tbsp garlic-infused oil
- 2 carrots, thinly sliced on the diagonal
- 1½ tbsp gluten-free plain (all-purpose) flour
- 3 tsp mild curry powder
- 600ml / 2½ cups gluten-free chicken stock
- 4 tsp gluten-free soy sauce
- 2 bay leaves
- 1 tsp garam masala

Here's another one that I always used to watch Mark eat in envy. Who wouldn't crave golden, crispy chicken with a warming, mildly spicy curry sauce and sticky rice? You can always cheat and serve up the sauce with gluten-free breadcrumbed chicken from the supermarket too. Give it a try my way first though – trust me, it's worth it!

Preheat the oven to 200°C fan / 220°C / 425°F.

To prepare your chicken breasts, butterfly them carefully, using a sharp knife. If you're not familiar with this technique, it might be easier to place the chicken breasts between two sheets of cling film (plastic wrap) and bash until flat with a rolling pin or meat mallet. Either way, aim to make the chicken breast as flat as possible.

Crack the egg into a small bowl and beat with a fork, then grab two large plates. On one plate, spread out the flour, and on the other spread out your breadcrumbs.

Dredge the chicken in the flour until well coated, then dip it into the beaten egg until coated. Finally, roll it around in the breadcrumbs until tightly covered.

Add your vegetable oil to a large pan so that it fully covers the base. Place over a medium heat and, once heated, gently place your breadcrumbed chicken in the oil – it should sizzle. Cook on each side for 2–3 minutes until almost golden, then place on a baking tray and cook in the oven for 10–12 minutes until golden and the chicken is cooked through.

Now for your katsu sauce. In a clean, large pan heat the garlic-infused oil over a medium heat. Fry the carrots for 2–3 minutes until slightly softened. Add the flour and curry powder, mix well until all the carrots are coated and continue to cook for 1 minute.

Add in your chicken stock, soy sauce and bay leaves. Bring to the boil, then turn down the heat and simmer for 20 minutes or until the sauce thickens. Once it is a nice, thick, yet still pourable consistency, stir in the garam masala. Remove from the heat and discard the bay leaves. Traditionally, you'd then strain the sauce to remove the carrots, but you can optionally leave these in too – they taste great!

Sprinkle with the chopped chives and serve with sticky jasmine rice.

Making it veggie?
Replace the chicken with veg like aubergine (eggplant), sweet potato and butternut squash cut into 1cm / ⅜in discs. Use gluten-free vegetable/vegan stock and continue the recipe as directed, bearing in mind that the veg might need a little longer in the oven.

Making it vegan?
Follow the steps above to make it veggie, but instead of using an egg to coat your veg before dipping them in breadcrumbs, mix 100ml / generous ⅓ cup soy milk with 2 tsp lemon juice. Allow to rest for 10 minutes before using.

Making it low FODMAP?
Use low FODMAP stock cube and breadcrumbs. Ensure the curry powder and garam masala are onion/garlic-free.

Korean-style FRIED CHICKEN TENDERS

ensure ketchup/ miso paste is onion/garlic-free

SERVES · 3-4

TAKES · 40 MINUTES

- 125g / 1¼ cups cornflour (cornstarch)
- 1 tsp salt
- 600g / 1lb 5oz chicken breast mini fillets
- 500ml / 2 cups vegetable oil
- Handful of roasted peanuts, chopped (ensure gluten-free)
- 2 tbsp sesame seeds
- Handful of spring onion (scallion) greens, shredded (optional)

For the sauce

- 60ml / ¼ cup gluten-free soy sauce
- 150ml / ⅝ cup maple syrup
- 1 tsp dried chilli flakes
- 1 tsp minced ginger paste
- 1 tsp miso paste (ensure gluten-free)
- 1 tbsp tomato ketchup
- 1 tbsp rice wine vinegar
- 1 tbsp garlic-infused oil
- 1 tbsp cornflour (cornstarch)
- 2 tbsp cold water

Here's the other kind of 'KFC' we can never eat. Think super crunchy, fried chicken in a thick, sticky, sweet and spicy sauce. One bite and you'll be hooked!

In a large mixing bowl, mix your cornflour with the salt. Add your chicken fillets and toss until well coated, squeezing the chicken and compacting the flour to it as much as you can.

Grab a large, heavy-based saucepan and pour in the vegetable oil until it is about 2.5cm / 1in deep. Place over a medium heat until the oil reaches 170°C / 340°F; test the temperature with a cooking thermometer, or by using the wooden spoon handle test (page 19). In 2 batches, carefully lower your coated chicken into the oil – it should sizzle nicely.

Cook for around 5 minutes or until the crispy coating starts to turn golden – if your oil covers all of your chicken, you shouldn't need to turn it. Remove with a slotted spoon and transfer to a wire rack set over a baking tray to drain.

Once all the chicken is done, refry in 2 batches in the oil for another 4-5 minutes. This is the key to making them super crunchy so don't skip this bit! Remove and transfer back to the wire rack to drain once more.

For the sauce, combine everything except the cornflour and water in a large wok. Bring to the boil and allow to simmer for 4-5 minutes. Mix the cornflour and water together in a small dish, drizzle into the wok and stir in immediately. Simmer until the sauce thickens. Finally, add the peanuts and your crunchy fried chicken to the wok, mix until everything is well coated, sprinkle with sesame seeds and shredded spring onion then serve immediately.

Serve up with my egg-fried rice (page 93).

Making it veggie? Or vegan? Use a block of extra-firm tofu in place of the chicken, cut into wide, thin strips, and proceed with the recipe as directed, halving the cooking time.

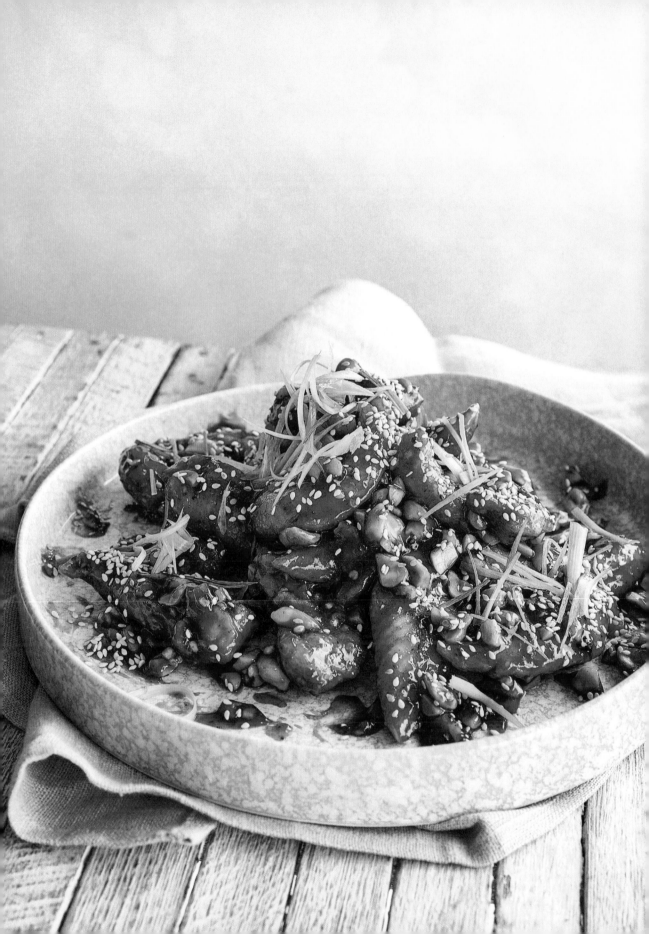

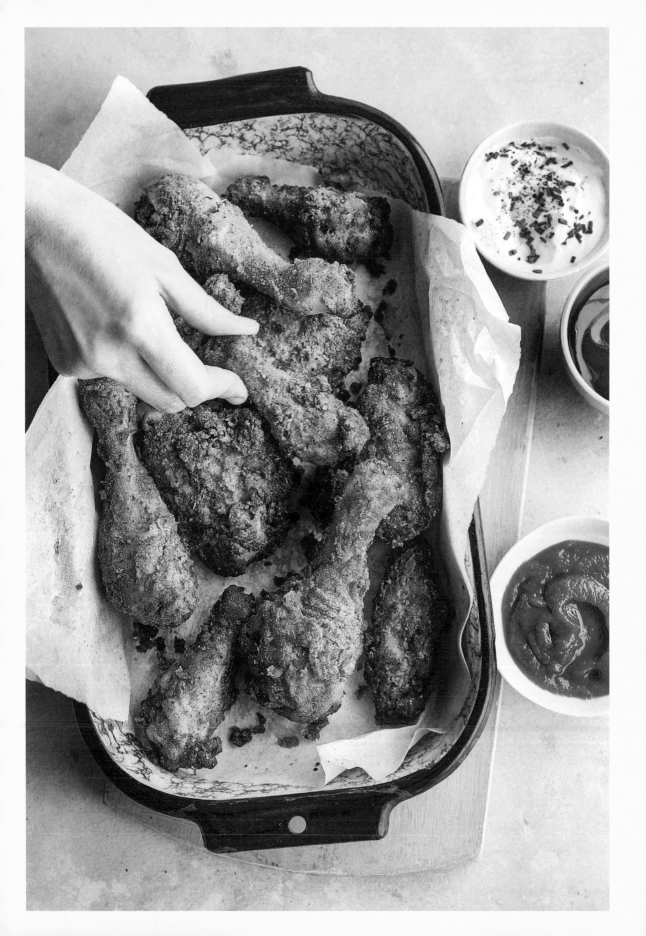

Gluten-free KFC

SERVES · 4

TAKES · 45 MINUTES + 30 MINUTES CHILLING

- 1kg / 2lb 2oz chicken thighs, drumsticks or wings, bone in, skin on (feel free to use chicken breast mini fillets or chicken tenders)
- 285ml / scant 1¼ cups buttermilk
- 1.5l / 6½ cups vegetable oil

For the coating

- 230g / 1¾ cups gluten-free plain (all-purpose) flour
- 2 tsp dried thyme
- 2 tsp dried basil
- 1½ tsp dried oregano
- 1 tbsp celery salt
- 1 tbsp dried mustard
- 2 tbsp smoked paprika
- 1 tbsp ground ginger
- 2 tbsp white pepper

I haven't been into a KFC in over a decade, for obvious reasons. I think I could probably only eat a napkin! My new and improved recipe is based on the 'leaked' KFC recipe that was posted online a few years ago. After a little tweaking, I've got it to the point where it genuinely tastes like the real deal.

Put your chicken and buttermilk into a large bowl and mix until well coated. Cover and chill for at least 30 minutes, but ideally overnight in the fridge (return the chicken to room temperature before cooking, if possible).

Heat the oil in a deep, heavy-based saucepan over a medium heat for about 15 minutes, until it reaches 170°C / 340°F, making sure the pan is not more than half full, as the oil will bubble up when cooking. Test the temperature with a cooking thermometer, or by using the wooden spoon handle test (page 19).

Meanwhile, mix together all of your coating ingredients in a large bowl and spread out on a large plate. Take the chicken pieces out of the buttermilk and roll them in the seasoned flour until all sides are well coated.

Once the oil has heated, take three pieces of chicken at a time and carefully lower into the oil. Cook drumsticks and thighs for 10–12 minutes; wings and chicken breast strips should take around 10 minutes. Once cooked, remove from the oil with a slotted spoon and place onto a wire rack set over a baking tray to drain while you cook the remaining chicken pieces.

Serve immediately with all your favourite sides – we love it with coleslaw, mashed potatoes and gravy. Or if you're feeling adventurous, serve up on top of my gluten-free waffles (page 69).

TIP:

If you can tolerate onion and garlic, you can also add 1 tsp each of garlic powder and onion powder to the coating seasoning.

Making it dairy-free?
Make your own buttermilk by combining 285ml / scant 1¼ cups soy milk with 3 tbsp lemon juice. Allow to rest for 10 minutes and continue with the recipe as directed.

Making it lactose-free? Or low FODMAP?
Make your own buttermilk by combining 285ml / scant 1¼ cups lactose-free milk with 3 tbsp lemon juice. Allow to rest for 10 minutes and continue with the recipe as directed.

Making it veggie? Or vegan?
Follow the advice above to make this dairy-free and use king oyster mushrooms instead of chicken, chopped into nice, thick, meaty chunks. Continue with the recipe as directed.

Pizza Margherita

THIN & CRISPY OR DEEP-PAN

dairy free

use dairy-free cheese

vegetarian

vegan

low lactose

MAKES · 2 THIN BASES OR 1 DEEP-PAN

TAKES · 25 MINUTES

- 1 quantity of gluten-free pizza dough (page 47)
- Gluten-free plain (all-purpose) flour, for dusting

For the tomato sauce

- 150ml / ⅝ cup passata (sieved tomatoes)
- 1 tsp garlic-infused oil
- 1 tbsp dried oregano
- Salt and pepper

For the toppings

- 125g / 4oz mozzarella cheese, thinly sliced
- Fresh basil leaves

I find it hard to believe that I went so long without eating pizza. Especially when it's so incredibly simple to make at home using my 3-ingredient gluten-free pizza dough! You can either make two thin and crispy style pizzas or one deep-pan pizza, depending on how thick you roll out your dough. But best of all, nobody would ever even know that it's gluten-free. Add whatever toppings you like.

Take your gluten-free pizza dough, having rested it for 30 minutes, and place on a lightly floured surface.

For two thin and crispy pizzas, cut the dough ball in half. Use a floured rolling pin to roll out your dough portion to a 5mm / ¼in thickness. For one deep-pan pizza, roll out your entire dough to a 1cm / ⅜in thickness. Aim for a nice, round shape that'll fit into your (large) frying pan; I find it easiest to roll the dough a little bigger than my frying pan, then cut around the base of the frying pan to ensure it fits perfectly. If the edges are a little cracked, simply use your fingers to gently shape them until smooth.

Place the frying pan over a high heat. Once hot, carefully transfer your dough into the dry pan, using a cake lifter or pizza peel.

Cook on one side for 2 minutes, then flip and cook for a further 1 minute. After flipping, press down firmly using a spatula – this encourages the base to puff up a little. Repeat using the other half of your dough, if making two.

Preheat the oven to 200°C fan / 220°C / 425°F.

Combine all the sauce ingredients in a small bowl, with salt and pepper to taste. Spread the sauce onto your base, leaving a 1cm / ⅜in gap for the crust. Next, top your pizza with lots of thinly sliced mozzarella. At this point you can add whatever toppings you like – it's totally up to you.

Bake in the oven, either on a pizza tray, or straight onto the oven shelf, for 8-10 minutes until the cheese is nicely browned and golden. Finish with some basil leaves, slice and serve immediately.

TIP:
These are freezer-friendly! After you've fried the pizza bases on both sides, they can then be frozen. The next time you fancy a pizza, simply top the frozen bases and cook for an extra couple of minutes.

Making it low FODMAP?
Use no more than 40g / 1½oz of mozzarella per person. If making 1 deep pan pizza, only use half of the tomato sauce.

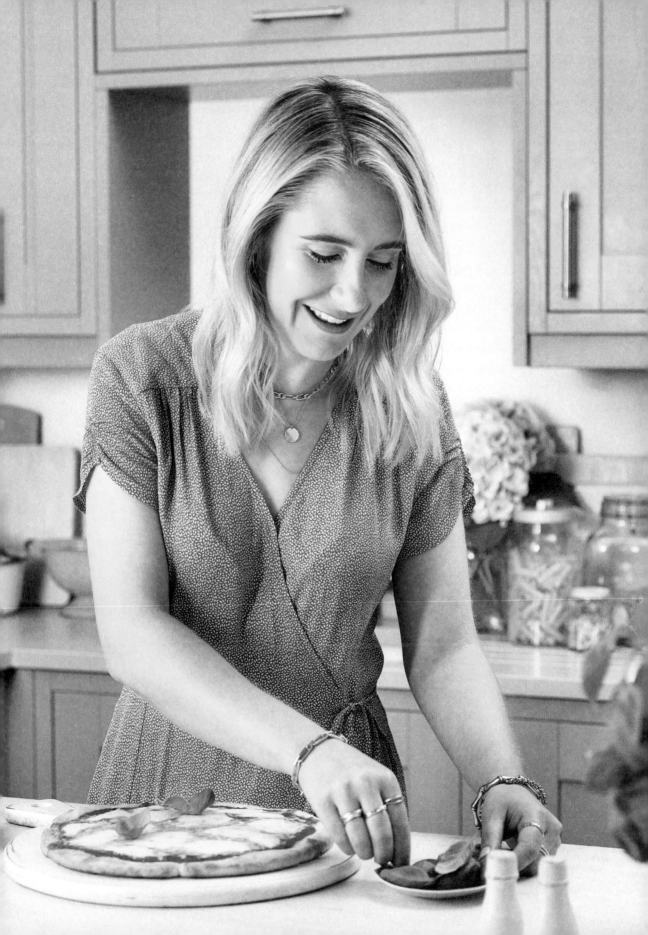

Thin and Crispy
Margherita

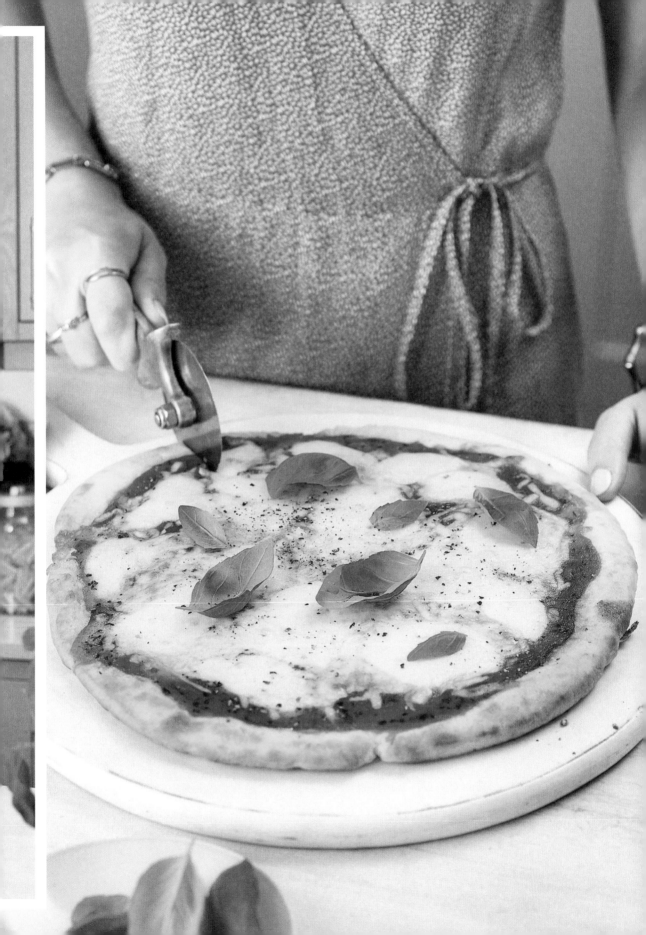

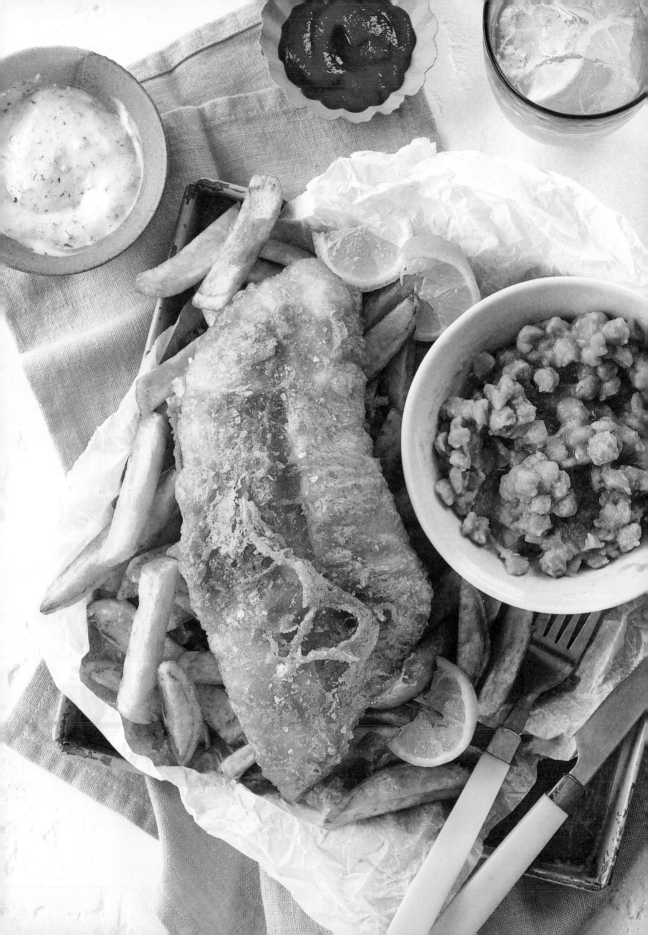

Beer-battered FISH & CHIPS

SERVES · 2

TAKES · 45 MINUTES

- 1.5l / 6½ cups vegetable oil
- 4 medium potatoes
- 50g / 6 tbsp gluten-free plain (all-purpose) flour
- 2 white fish fillets, skinless (I recommend cod or haddock)

For the batter

- 110g / ¾ cup gluten-free plain (all-purpose) flour
- 2 tsp gluten-free baking powder
- 1 tsp salt
- 150ml / ⅝ cup gluten-free beer or carbonated water

Here's how to make beer-battered fish and chips at home that you'd never guess were gluten-free. In fact, you'd never guess it was homemade either! If your local chippy doesn't have a separate fryer for gluten-free food, then it's about time you made it at home.

Heat the oil in a deep, heavy-based saucepan over a medium heat for about 15 minutes, or until it reaches 170°C / 340°F, making sure the pan is not more than half full, as the oil will bubble up when cooking. Test the temperature with a cooking thermometer, or by using the wooden spoon handle test (page 19).

While the oil is heating, combine the dry ingredients for your batter in a large mixing bowl. Give it a mix and set aside.

Peel and cut the potatoes into 1cm / ½in thick chip shapes then pat dry with some kitchen paper. They need to be as dry as possible before frying to get them nice and crisp. Place to one side.

Grab a large plate and spread the flour out on it. Place your fish fillets on the plate and dust until lightly coated.

Once your oil is hot, add your chips and cook for 8 minutes, then remove them from the oil with a slotted spoon and place onto a wire rack set over a baking tray to drain.

Make sure your oil is still at 170°C / 340°F then add your gluten-free beer or carbonated water to the dry batter ingredients and whisk until consistent (it's important not to add this any sooner or it will lose its fizz).

Dredge your fish fillets in the batter mixture, then carefully lower each fillet, one at a time, into the oil. Cook for 7-8 minutes until the batter is golden and crispy, bearing in mind that using carbonated water makes it a little lighter in colour. Remove from the oil and place onto the wire rack set over a baking tray to drain.

Lastly, add your chips back into the hot oil and cook for around 3-4 minutes until golden. Allow to drain once more on the wire rack before serving with tartare sauce and mushy peas.

TIPS:
Long fillets of white fish work best here instead of smaller, chunky fillets, which are more prone to flaking apart when you pick them up and are harder to safely lower into hot oil. You can also use this batter to make your own homemade onion rings. I can't tolerate onion, so enjoy them for me!

Making it veggie?
Use thin strips of halloumi instead of white fish. Ensure your gluten-free beer is vegetarian too.

Making it vegan?
Instead of using white fish, simply substitute with canned banana blossom (drained). Just pull off any stringy bits, pat dry with kitchen paper and proceed with the recipe as directed. Ensure your gluten-free beer is vegan too.

DIY
Doner Kebab

SERVES · 2-3

TAKES · 45 MINUTES

- 250g / 9oz minced (ground) lamb
- 250g / 9oz minced (ground) beef
- 1 tsp ground cumin
- 1 tsp smoked paprika
- 1 tsp ground coriander
- 1 tbsp dried mixed herbs
- 3 tbsp garlic-infused oil
- 1 large egg
- 1 tsp salt
- Generous pinch of pepper

For the herby garlic sauce (optional)

- 100ml / scant ½ cup mayonnaise
- 1½ tsp garlic-infused oil
- 1½ tsp dried mixed herbs

To serve

- 2-ingredient flatbreads (page 58)
- Salad of your choice

Whip up your own homemade doner kebab without having to worry about the nightmare that is cross-contamination. Feel free to use all lamb mince instead of the lamb/beef combo too. Using a food processor makes this quick and easy, but isn't mandatory. Eating this at 3am is optional, however!

Preheat the oven to 200°C fan / 220°C / 425°F.

If using a food processor, add all of your kebab ingredients and blend until smooth. If mixing by hand, add everything to a mixing bowl and mix with a wooden spoon until well combined, mashing the mixture as much as you can to ensure it's nice and smooth, without lumps.

Add your mixture to a 900g / 2lb loaf tin and compact it in. Cover the top with foil and bake in the oven for 20–25 minutes. Remove, then carefully turn out onto a plate and baste with the juices left in the loaf tin, leaving a little of the juice for later if you intend to do the last optional grilling (broiling) step.

Allow to rest for 15–20 minutes, if you have the time – that way, you'll get cleaner shavings off it. Once rested, take a sharp knife and shave off lots of super-thin slices.

If you like, place the shavings on a baking tray, baste with a little of the juice left in the loaf tin and grill (broil) for 10 minutes for a true doner kebab-like finish.

If serving with the herby garlic dip, mix the ingredients together in a small bowl.

Serve up the kebabs with my 2-ingredient flatbreads as well as salad and herby garlic dip.

TIP:
Using higher-fat-content mince will prevent the meat from drying out in the oven. If using lean mince, I'd recommend adding an extra egg.

Making it veggie? Or vegan?
Simply omit the egg and lamb / beef and fry 200g / 7oz shredded king oyster mushrooms in garlic-infused oil. Then add the spice blend used in this recipe. Serve up with the accompaniments suggested and use vegan mayo for the herby garlic sauce.

·ONE-POT BBQ·
Pulled Pork Tacos

 use lactose-free cheese

 use dairy-free cheese

SERVES · 4

**TAKES · 20 MINUTES
+ 2 HOURS 45 MINUTES
COOK TIME**

- 1kg / 2lb 2oz pork shoulder, boneless
- 2 tbsp garlic-infused oil
- 300ml / 1¼ cups (hard) cider (ensure gluten-free)

For the rub
- 2 tsp smoked paprika
- ½ tsp black pepper
- 1 tsp celery salt
- 3 tbsp dark brown sugar
- 1 tsp cayenne pepper (optional)

For the BBQ sauce
- 220ml / 1 cup tomato ketchup
- 2 tsp smoked paprika
- 1 tbsp black treacle (molasses)

To serve
- 2-ingredient corn tortillas (page 59)
- Baby gem lettuce, shredded
- Spring onion (scallion) greens, chopped
- Extra mature Cheddar cheese, grated

For me, street food usually involves walking down the street and taking in the combined aroma of all the food I *can't* eat. But as that isn't much of a hobby, I decided to make the ultimate street-food fakeaway of my dreams instead! This pulled pork is super soft and tender in the middle, yet crisp on the outside and packed with tons of sweet, smoky flavour. Add in the cayenne pepper if you like a little extra kick.

Preheat your oven to 150°C fan / 170°C / 340°F.

In a large mixing bowl, add all the ingredients for the rub and mix until well combined. Ensure you break up any large clumps of sugar. Add the pork shoulder to the bowl and, using your hands, cover completely with the rub. Squeeze it and compact it against the pork shoulder as much as possible.

Place a large lidded flameproof casserole dish or Dutch oven over a medium heat. Add your garlic-infused oil. Once hot, add the pork shoulder to the dish. Sear both sides and both ends for 1 minute each. Propping up the pork shoulder against the side of the dish can help when searing the ends. A carving fork is a great tool for easily turning that big hunk of pork!

Once the pork is seared on all sides, pour in your cider, pop the lid on and place into the preheated oven for 2½ hours. Once the 2½ hours is up, remove the lid and cook for a further 15-20 minutes.

Remove the pork from the dish and place onto a large plate. Allow to rest for 10 minutes.

To make your BBQ sauce, add the tomato ketchup, smoked paprika and black treacle to the casserole dish with all the meat juices and cider (there should be approximately 230ml / scant 1 cup of meat juice and cider). Stir everything together until fully combined.

Shred the rested pork using two forks. Add all of the shredded pork back into the casserole dish and mix into the BBQ sauce.

Serve up immediately with my 2-ingredient corn tortillas alongside shredded baby gem lettuce, chopped spring onion greens and grated Cheddar.

I also love to enjoy this pulled pork stuffed into brioche buns (page 46) or 2-ingredient arepas (page 60).

Making it low FODMAP?
Simply use gluten-free beer instead of cider and enjoy without the BBQ sauce, or serve with a low-FODMAP BBQ sauce instead.

HOME COMFORTS

This chapter is dedicated to all the meals I've enjoyed in the only place in the world where I can eat absolutely everything... my own home!

That includes all the meals I grew up eating with my mum, dad and little bro Charlie (who obviously now towers over me). As you might expect, all those meals back then contained gluten, so I've since adapted them all to be gluten-free. After all, how sad would it be if I never got to eat all those nostalgic meals that remind me of home?

The other side of home comforts for me is all the things that my boyfriend Mark and I have enjoyed since we moved in together. As Mark's mum is from Malaysia, that also includes his home comforts, which have now become mine too.

So this chapter is a real mix of easy-to-make meals that we'd probably cook for you if you came over for dinner. Take your shoes off at the door, please!

ONE-POT
Beef Stew
· & SUET DUMPLINGS

use a low
FODMAP
stock cube

SERVES · 3-4

**TAKES · 1 HOUR
30 MINUTES**

- 3 tbsp garlic-infused oil
- 400g / 14oz beef braising steak (chuck steak), cut into 2.5 x 1.5cm / 1 x ½in strips
- 1½ tbsp gluten-free plain (all-purpose) flour
- 1 medium carrot, peeled and chopped
- 1 medium parsnip, peeled and chopped
- 300g / 10½oz new potatoes, halved
- 400ml / 1⅔ cups gluten-free beef stock
- 100ml / generous ⅓ cup red wine (or add more beef stock)
- 1 bay leaf
- 1½ tbsp dried thyme
- Salt and pepper

For the dumplings

- 150g / generous 1 cup gluten-free plain (all-purpose) flour
- 1 tsp gluten-free baking powder
- 80g / 3oz gluten-free vegetable suet
- 2 tbsp dried thyme (optional)
- Pinch of salt
- 95ml / 6 tbsp water

This hearty, warming stew is packed with tender beef and veg that soak up all that rich, thick gravy. Of course, what would a beef stew be without those lovely soft yet stodgy suet dumplings on top? We always throw potatoes into the pot to make this an easy all-in-one meal.

Preheat your oven to 180°C fan / 200°C / 400°F.

In a large Dutch oven or lidded flameproof casserole dish, add your garlic-infused oil and place over a medium heat. Add the beef and stir-fry for 3-4 minutes until browned on all sides.

Sprinkle in the flour and stir so that the beef is completely coated. Immediately add your carrot, parsnip and potatoes, stir and fry for another 1-2 minutes. Pour in your stock, red wine then add the bay leaf and thyme. Season with a little salt and pepper, pop the lid on and cook in the oven for 50 minutes.

Meanwhile, prepare your dumplings. Add all the dry ingredients to a large mixing bowl and slowly add the water, mixing it in until it forms a thick dough. Too sticky? Add a little more flour. Too dry? Add a little extra water.

Divide the dough into 6 equal balls, then place back in the mixing bowl, cover and set aside. After 50 minutes, take the dish out of the oven and remove the lid, then arrange the dumplings over the stew, submerging them so that just the tops are visible. Pop the lid back on and place in the oven for a further 10 minutes, then remove the lid and cook for a final 20 minutes.

Don't forget to remove the bay leaf before serving!

TIPS:
Can't find gluten-free vegetable suet for the dumplings? Use 80g / ⅓ cup cold butter or hard margarine and rub into the dry ingredients before adding water. You can also make this with skinless, boneless chicken thighs instead of beef.

Making it veggie? Or vegan?
Replace the beef with an equal amount of sweet potato, peeled and chopped into chunks. Use a gluten-free vegetable/vegan stock cube and ensure the red wine is vegetarian/vegan.

ONE-POT
Campfire Stew

SERVES · 2

TAKES · 30 MINUTES

- 3 tbsp garlic-infused oil
- 400g / 14oz gluten-free pork sausages
- 1 carrot, thinly sliced
- 1 yellow (bell) pepper, chopped
- 1 tbsp dried mixed herbs
- 1 tbsp smoked paprika
- ½ tsp ground cumin
- ½ tsp dried chilli flakes
- ½ tsp black pepper
- 1 tbsp gluten-free plain (all-purpose) flour
- 1 tsp gluten-free Worcestershire sauce (optional)
- 250ml / 1 cup water
- 1 x 400g / 14oz can chopped tomatoes
- ½ gluten-free beef or ham stock cube
- 125g / ¾ cup canned butter beans (lima beans), drained
- Handful of spring onion (scallion) greens, chopped

While a regular stew would take well over an hour, you can throw this one together in just 30 minutes. It's hearty, warming, mildly spicy, with meaty sausages and tender veg that soak up all that marvellous flavour. Plus, there's only one pot to wash up afterwards!

In a large Dutch oven or lidded flameproof casserole dish, add your garlic-infused oil and place over a medium-high heat. Add your sausages and fry for 5 minutes until lightly browned. Then add your carrot and yellow pepper and stir-fry for 4–5 minutes.

Add in the herbs and spices, the flour and the Worcestershire sauce, if using, and stir for 2 minutes until everything is well coated. Add the water and chopped tomatoes then crumble in the half stock cube.

Bring to the boil and simmer for 20 minutes or until the veg is cooked and the stew is lovely and thick. Stir in the butter beans and cook for a further 5 minutes.

Lastly, throw in the spring onion greens and serve immediately, with a chunky slice of buttered gluten-free white bread (page 41) or my gluten-free flatbreads (page 58).

Making it veggie? Or vegan?
Replace the pork sausages with gluten-free meat-alternative sausages and use a gluten-free vegetable/vegan stock cube instead.

Making it low FODMAP?
Use a low FODMAP stock cube and only add 70g / ½ cup butter beans. Ensure the sausages don't contain onion or garlic. The low FODMAP serving size is just under a quarter of the entire finished stew. Omit Worcestershire sauce.

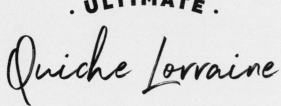

· ULTIMATE ·
Quiche Lorraine

use a dairy-free milk, cheese and cream alternative

use lactose-free cream/milk

use lactose-free cream/milk

SERVES · 4-6

TAKES · 1 HOUR 20 MINUTES

- 1 quantity of gluten-free shortcrust pastry (page 27), chilled for 25 minutes
- Gluten-free plain (all-purpose) flour, for dusting
- 120ml / ½ cup milk
- 200ml / generous ¾ cup double (heavy) cream
- 3 eggs
- 200g / 7oz smoked streaky bacon, grilled or fried, then diced
- 100g / 3½oz extra mature Cheddar cheese, grated
- Salt and pepper

Once your shortcrust pastry is prepared, you're only 5 simple ingredients away from a quiche like no other. With beautifully buttery pastry filled with smoky bacon and a creamy, cheesy egg filling, you'll have to fight the muggles away from this one!

Remove your pastry from the fridge. If it feels really firm, leave it out at room temperature briefly. Don't handle your dough excessively as this will warm it up and make it more fragile.

Lightly flour your rolling pin. On a sheet of non-stick baking parchment, roll out the dough to a large circle, 2mm / ⅟₁₆in thick. Transfer the pastry to a 23cm / 9in fluted tart tin (pan), by supporting the pastry as you gently invert it into the tin, with equal overhang on all sides. Peel off the baking parchment.

Next, use your fingers to carefully ease the pastry into place so that it neatly lines the tin. Lift the overhanging pastry and, using your thumb, squash 2mm / ⅟₁₆in of pastry back into the tin. This will result in slightly thicker sides, which will prevent your pastry case from shrinking when baked. Allow the remaining overhang to do its thing – we'll trim it after chilling it.

Lightly prick the base of the pastry case with a fork and place in the fridge for 15 minutes. Preheat the oven to 180°C fan / 200°C / 400°F and place a large baking tray in the oven to heat up.

After chilling, use a rolling pin to roll over the top of the tin, removing the pastry overhang. Loosely line the base of the pastry case with baking parchment and fill with baking beans (or uncooked rice if you don't have any). Place the tin onto the heated baking tray in the oven and cook for 15 minutes. Remove the baking parchment and baking beans, then bake for a further 5 minutes.

Meanwhile, in a large jug (pitcher), beat together the milk, cream and eggs, then season generously with salt and pepper. Remove the pastry case and baking tray from the oven and work quickly from this point so the baking tray doesn't lose its heat.

Spread the crispy bacon and three-quarters of your grated cheese evenly across the base of the pastry case. Pour the egg mixture into the pastry case, then top with your reserved cheese. Carefully place back in the oven (ensuring you don't spill any!), still on the hot baking tray, and cook for 30 minutes. Once cooked, it should look lovely and golden brown on top, a little risen and not 'jiggly'.

Allow to cool for 5 minutes before removing from the tin and serving warm with a rocket (arugula) salad.

TIP:
If you don't have time to make your own pastry, use store-bought gluten-free pastry instead.

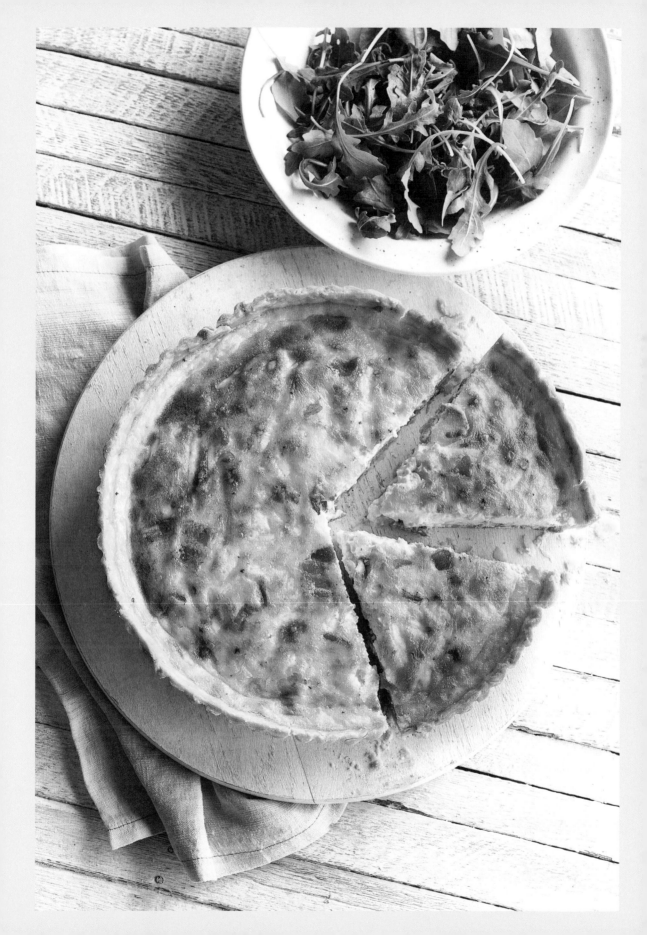

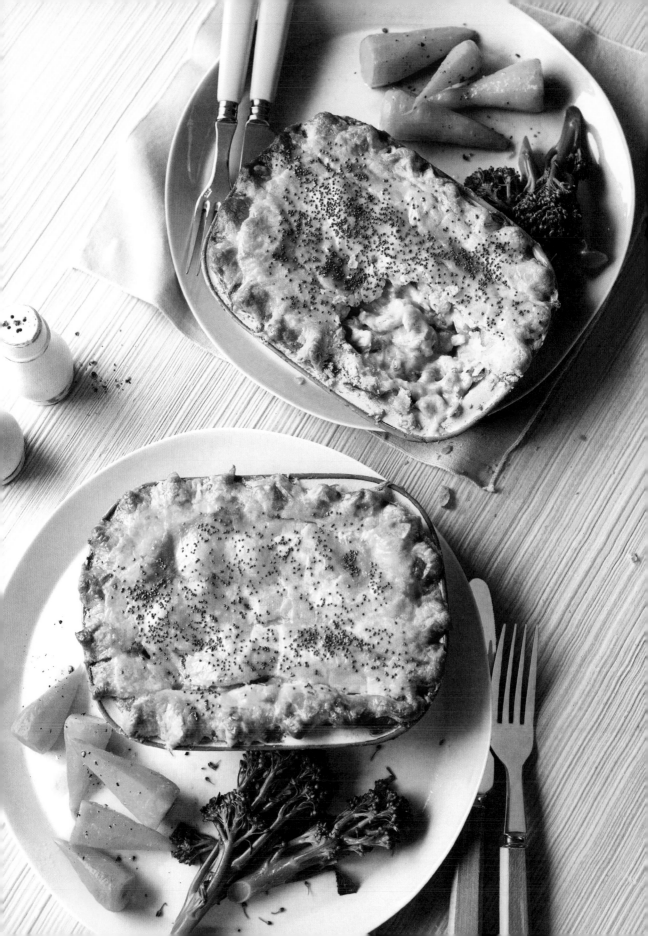

Mini
CHICKEN, LEEK AND BACON *Pies*

 use a dairy-free cream alternative

 use lactose-free cream, the green parts of the leek only and a low FODMAP stock cube

 use lactose-free cream

MAKES · 2

TAKES · 45 MINUTES

- 1 quantity of gluten-free shortcrust pastry (page 27), chilled for 25 minutes
- 1 egg, beaten
- Handful of poppy seeds (optional)

For the filling

- 250g / 9oz boneless, skinless chicken thigh fillets
- 100g / 3½oz smoked streaky bacon, diced
- 90g / 3¼oz leek, chopped
- 2 tbsp gluten-free plain (all-purpose) flour, plus extra for dusting
- 400ml / 1⅔ cups gluten-free chicken stock
- Sprig of fresh rosemary, finely chopped
- 2 tbsp double (heavy) cream
- Salt and pepper

With tons of creamy, chunky filling encased in buttery pastry, I'm in love with these cute little, single-serve pies. At home, I use two 10cm / 4in round ceramic pie dishes to make these but if making one large pie, you'll need to double the quantity of pastry and multiply the filling ingredients by 1.5.

For the filling, cut the chicken into small strips no more than 2cm / ¾in long. Place a large pan over a medium heat, add your bacon and fry until the fat begins to brown, then add your leek and chicken strips. Fry for 3–4 minutes, occasionally stirring, until the chicken is sealed.

Add in your flour and mix until everything is evenly coated, then add the stock and rosemary, and season with salt and pepper. Bring to the boil and simmer for 10 minutes or until the gravy has nicely thickened. Remove from the heat and, after 5 minutes, stir in the cream and leave to cool.

Preheat your oven to 200°C fan / 220°C / 425°F.

Remove your pastry from the fridge – if it feels really firm when you take it out, leave it out at room temperature briefly. Don't handle your dough excessively as this will warm it up and make it more fragile. Cut the ball of pastry in half and lightly flour your rolling pin. On a sheet of non-stick baking parchment, roll out one portion of the dough to a 3mm / ⅛in thickness.

If using a round 10cm / 4in pie dish, cut out a 12cm / 4¾in circle from your rolled-out pastry. Transfer this to a pie dish and gently push the pastry in, using your fingers, leaving a little overhang, but trimming

off any excess that hangs down over the edge of the dish. If using a rectangular pie dish, ensure that you have rolled your pastry into a rectangular shape, then simply transfer the pastry to the pie dish as above, trimming any excess.

Form the leftover pastry scraps back into a ball and reroll out to a 3mm / ⅛in thickness. Place your second pie dish face down onto the rolled-out pastry and trace around it with a knife to create a lid. Place the lid to one side (you'll need to trace around it with a knife to make the second lid later). Repeat with the other half of your dough and second pie dish.

Divide your pie filling between the pie dishes and brush the overhang with egg. Place your pastry lids on top and pinch the edges together to crimp them tightly shut.

Brush each pie with beaten egg and sprinkle with poppy seeds, if you like. Lastly, make a small hole in the very middle of the top of each lid by gently prodding with a sharp knife and twisting. Cook in the oven for 30 minutes until golden, then serve with mashed potato, veggies and my lazy gluten-free gravy (page 33).

TIP:
If you don't have time to make your own pastry, use store-bought gluten-free pastry instead.

Mum's
EASY LASAGNE

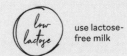

low lactose

use lactose-free milk

SERVES · 6

TAKES · 1 HOUR 20 MINUTES

For the ragu

- 3 tbsp garlic-infused oil
- 1 carrot, diced
- 1 celery stick, diced (optional)
- 750g / 1lb 10oz minced (ground) beef
- 200ml / generous ¾ cup red wine (or beef stock)
- 2 x 400g / 14oz cans chopped tomatoes
- 2 tbsp tomato purée (paste)
- 2 tbsp dried mixed herbs
- 2 handfuls of spring onion (scallion) greens, chopped (optional)
- Salt and pepper

For the white sauce

- 50g / 3½ tbsp butter
- 50g / 6 tbsp gluten-free plain (all-purpose) flour
- 750ml / 3 cups milk
- 75g / 2¾oz extra mature Cheddar cheese, grated
- 2 tsp wholegrain mustard (optional)
- Salt and pepper

To assemble

- 10–12 gluten-free lasagne sheets (page 24 or store-bought)
- 20g / ¾oz extra mature Cheddar cheese, grated
- Fresh basil (optional)

Crammed with layers of creamy white sauce, tender beef and perfectly cooked pasta, I have to say a big thank you to my mum for always making this gluten-free for me. My mum swears by an all-in-one method for the white sauce which makes it so much easier to make in a hurry.

Heat the garlic-infused oil in a large pan over a medium heat. Stir-fry the carrot and celery, if using, for 3–4 minutes. Add the minced beef and continue to fry for another 5 minutes or until all of it is nicely browned. Season with a little salt and pepper.

Pour in the wine or stock – if using wine, simmer for 5 minutes. Pour in the chopped tomatoes, followed by the tomato purée and mixed herbs. Bring to the boil and simmer for around 30 minutes until the sauce has thickened. Stir in your spring onion greens, if using, then remove from the heat.

Preheat the oven to 200°C fan / 220°C / 425°F.

For the white sauce, add the butter, flour and milk to a saucepan and place over a low heat. Immediately begin stirring with a wooden spoon and do not stop until it has transformed into a lovely, thick sauce. As you stir, make sure you keep scraping the bottom of the pan, otherwise the flour will sit there and become lumpy. Remove from the heat and throw in the grated cheese and mustard, if using. Season with a little salt and pepper to taste.

Now it's time to construct the lasagne. Grab a baking dish, about 30 x 20cm / 12 x 8in, and layer in the ragu, white sauce, then lasagne sheets, then repeat with another layer of each. Finish with a final layer of white sauce, making sure you don't leave any gaps. Finally, sprinkle the cheese over the top and bake in the oven for 30–40 minutes until golden brown on top.

Scatter with some fresh basil, if you like, and serve up with my gluten-free garlic bread pizza on page 92.

Making it dairy-free?
Use a good dairy-free cheese that melts well. For the white sauce, use dairy-free milk and a butter alternative.

Making it veggie?
Replace the beef with 2 diced courgettes (zucchini) and 1 diced aubergine (eggplant). If using red wine, ensure it is vegetarian or use gluten-free vegetable stock instead.

Making it vegan?
Combine the veggie and dairy-free advice above. Ensure the red wine is vegan, if using, or use vegan stock instead.

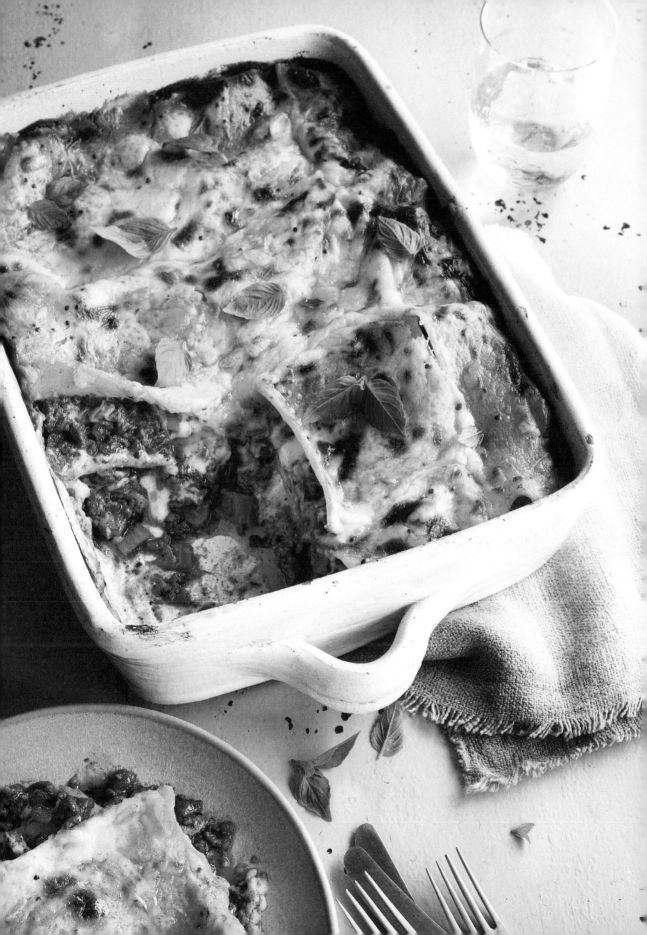

Lazy PEPPERONI GNOCCHI BAKE

 use dairy-free cheese

SERVES · 2–3

TAKES · 40 MINUTES

- 2 tbsp garlic-infused oil
- 1 yellow (bell) pepper, chopped
- 400g / 14oz gluten-free gnocchi (page 26 or store-bought)
- 1 tbsp smoked paprika
- 1 x 400g / 14oz can chopped tomatoes
- Handful of spring onion (scallion) greens, chopped, plus extra (optional) to finish
- 1 tsp dried mixed herbs
- 1 tsp sugar (optional)
- ½ tsp dried chilli flakes (optional)
- 125g / 4½oz mozzarella cheese (or buffalo mozzarella), thinly sliced
- 40g / 1½oz pepperoni
- Salt and pepper

Gnocchi is probably one of the easiest things you can make, but everyone always asks me what to do with it… so here you go! The sauce is lovely and smoky thanks to the smoked paprika, and the cheesy pepperoni top gives it that awesome pizza-like finish. This recipe only involves 10 minutes of effort and 20–30 minutes in the oven!

Preheat the oven to 200°C fan / 220°C / 425°F.

Heat the garlic-infused oil in a large pan or skillet over a medium heat, add the yellow pepper and stir-fry for 2 minutes, then add your gnocchi, followed by the smoked paprika, and stir-fry for another 3–4 minutes, ensuring all of the gnocchi is evenly coated.

Next, add in your chopped tomatoes, spring onion greens, mixed herbs, sugar and chilli flakes, if using, with salt and pepper to taste. Simmer for 5 minutes until the tomatoes have broken down.

If you're not using an ovenproof skillet, pour the contents of your pan into an ovenproof dish and spread the gnocchi and sauce out into a thin layer. If using an ovenproof skillet, just spread everything out in the skillet in an even layer.

Top with the mozzarella followed by the pepperoni and cook in the oven for 20–30 minutes until the mozzarella is nice and golden.

Finish with a little more chopped spring onion if you like, and serve up with my gluten-free garlic bread pizza (page 92).

Making it veggie?
Top with thinly sliced aubergine (eggplant) discs instead of pepperoni.

Making it vegan?
Use a good dairy-free cheese that melts well. Top with thinly sliced aubergine discs instead of pepperoni. If using store-bought gnocchi ensure that it is vegan.

Making it low FODMAP?
Use onion/garlic-free pepperoni, or smoky bacon if you can't find any. The low FODMAP serving size is just under a quarter of the entire finished gnocchi bake.

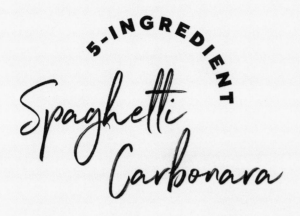

5-INGREDIENT
Spaghetti Carbonara

 use dairy-free cheese

SERVES · 2

TAKES · 15 MINUTES

- 200g / 7oz gluten-free spaghetti (store-bought or see page 24 to make tagliatelle)
- 3 eggs
- 60g / 2oz pecorino cheese, grated, plus extra to serve
- 1 tbsp garlic-infused oil
- 100g / 3½oz pancetta, diced
- Salt and black pepper

Who knew that you could make a proper spaghetti carbonara in 15 minutes with 5 ingredients? I've had carbonara many times before, but I still say that I didn't have my first 'real' carbonara until I had it in Rome. So I decided to recreate it at home! It's insanely creamy with little intense bites of pancetta throughout. *Bellissimo*!

If using store-bought spaghetti, cook according to the packet instructions, reserving a couple of tablespoons of the cooking water when you drain it. Gluten-free pasta can often clump together, but adding a teaspoon each of oil and salt to the water can massively help to prevent this.

While your pasta is cooking, crack your eggs into a jug (pitcher) and add in your grated cheese. Season with salt and plenty of pepper then beat with a fork until combined.

Heat the garlic-infused oil in a large pan over a medium heat. Add your pancetta and fry for 4–5 minutes or until it starts to crisp up, then turn the heat down to low.

Add your drained spaghetti to the pan and coat it evenly in all the oil and pancetta fat in the pan. Remove from the heat and add in your reserved 2 tablespoons of pasta cooking water, then pour in your egg and cheese mixture. Making sure you keep moving the egg mixture around, toss the spaghetti to coat it evenly. It's important to do this off the heat or your eggs will scramble!

Finish with a little more pepper and grated cheese on top and serve immediately.

TIP:
You can actually use whatever hard cheese you like – we often use Parmesan or extra mature Cheddar. Oh, and if you like your carbonara a little more 'saucy', use 100g / 3½oz pecorino cheese and an extra egg.

Making it veggie?
Replace the pancetta with 1 diced courgette (zucchini).

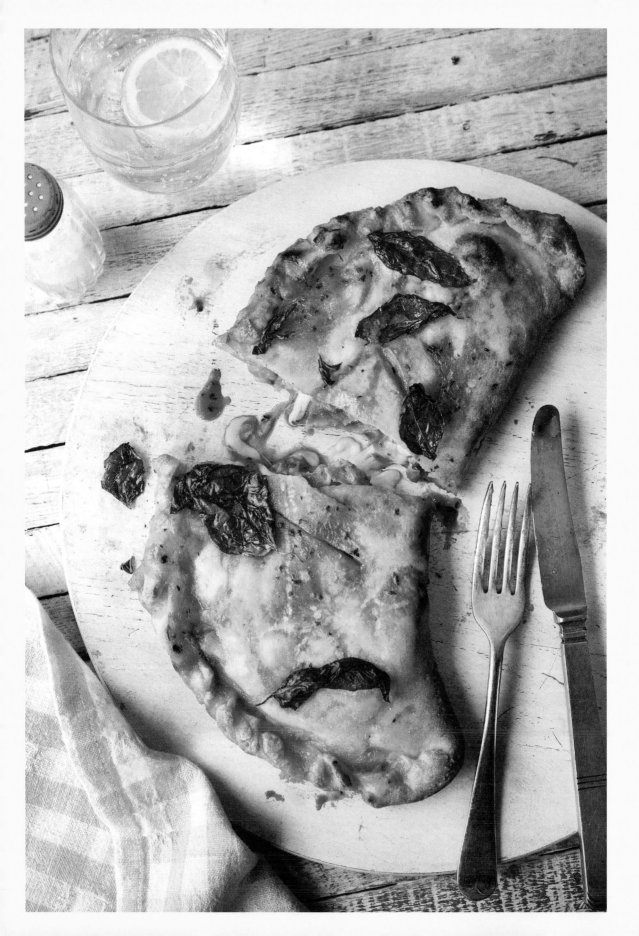

CHEESE & HAM
Calzone

 dairy-free — use dairy-free cheese

 low lactose

 vegan — use dairy-free cheese, omit the egg and use sautéed mushrooms instead of ham

 low fodmap

 vegetarian — use sautéed mushrooms instead of ham

SERVES · 3

TAKES · 25 MINUTES

- 1 quantity of gluten-free pizza dough (page 47)
- Gluten-free plain (all-purpose) flour, for dusting
- 1 egg, beaten
- Fresh basil (optional)

For the pizza sauce
- 100ml / generous ⅓ cup passata (sieved tomatoes)
- 1 tsp dried oregano
- ½ tsp garlic-infused oil
- Salt and black pepper

For the filling
- 120g / 4oz mozzarella cheese, thinly sliced
- Handful of fresh basil leaves
- 50g / 1¾oz prosciutto
- 2 tsp garlic-infused oil

I genuinely believed it was impossible to make an *edible* gluten-free calzone until I ate one (ok, about six) in Rome. With crispy pizza dough concealing an explosion of cheese and prosciutto, it's not only possible, it's so simple and quick too.

Preheat your oven to 240°C fan / 260°C / 500°F (or as hot as your oven will go if it doesn't reach these temperatures).

Grab a small bowl and mix together the ingredients for the pizza sauce, seasoning with a little salt and pepper to taste.

Take your pizza dough, having rested it for 30 minutes, and place on a lightly floured surface. Cut the dough into 2–3 pieces, depending on how many calzones you'd like to make and what size you'd prefer them. Using a rolling pin, roll each dough portion out to a rough circle, 4mm / ⅛in thick.

In the bottom third of your rolled-out dough, add a layer of mozzarella, followed by a few basil leaves, some prosciutto, 2–3 tablespoons of pizza sauce and a drizzle of garlic-infused oil, leaving a 2cm / ¾in gap between the filling and the edge of the dough. Brush the edges of your dough lightly with a little water to help it stick together.

Fold over the empty side of your dough so that it's 5mm / ⅛in short of meeting the edge of your filled side. It should form a neat semi-circle shape. Trim off any untidy edges using a pizza cutter.

Crimp the edge of your calzones shut by folding and pinching multiple times, all along the edge of the seam. Transfer to a baking tray lined with non-stick baking parchment. Brush all over with beaten egg then spoon another 1½ tablespoons of your pizza sauce on top of each calzone, gently spreading it using the back of the spoon. Top with a few basil leaves, if you like.

Finally, use a sharp knife to cut 3 slits into each calzone - this will allow steam to escape when cooking. Bake in the oven for 10 minutes until golden and crisp and serve up with rocket (arugula).

TIP:
We often use pepperoni or canned tuna instead of prosciutto - remix this recipe however you like!

Triple Cheese
MAC AND CHEESE

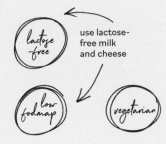

lactose free → use lactose-free milk and cheese

low fodmap

vegetarian

SERVES · 2

TAKES · 30 MINUTES

- 200g / 7oz gluten-free macaroni
- 2 tbsp garlic-infused oil
- 1 tbsp smoked paprika
- 1 tbsp gluten-free plain (all-purpose) flour
- 200ml / generous ¾ cup milk
- 75g / 3oz extra mature Cheddar cheese, grated
- 25g / 1oz pecorino cheese, grated
- 50g / 1¾oz mozzarella cheese, thinly sliced
- ½ tsp salt
- ½ tsp black pepper
- Handful of fresh chives, chopped, to serve

For the crispy top
- 50g / ⅔ cup gluten-free breadcrumbs (page 32 or store-bought)
- 1 tbsp dried mixed herbs

Yep, that's right. I said triple cheese. This cheese trilogy is the definition of comfort food and something you'll never see as a gluten-free option out in the wild. I'm absolutely in love with the stringy-ness that the mozzarella adds to the sauce combined with the crunch from that crispy, herby breadcrumb top.

Preheat your oven to 200°C fan / 220°C / 425°F.

Cook your macaroni according to the packet instructions. Gluten-free pasta can often clump together, but adding a teaspoon each of oil and salt to the water can massively help to prevent this.

While your pasta is cooking, place a large skillet or pan over a medium heat and add your garlic-infused oil. Once heated, add your smoked paprika and flour and whisk together for 1 minute until it forms a smooth paste. Pour in your milk and whisk constantly for 5 minutes until it forms a nice, smooth sauce. Take off the heat.

Add in your grated cheddar, pecorino and sliced mozzarella and mix until it all melts in, and the sauce is smooth, but slightly stringy. Stir in the salt and pepper. Add your drained macaroni and mix until well coated in the sauce.

If you're not using a skillet, pour the contents of your pan into an ovenproof dish and spread out into a thin layer. If using a skillet, just spread everything out in an even layer.

In a small bowl, combine your breadcrumbs and mixed herbs, sprinkle this over the top and cook in the oven for 15 minutes or until the breadcrumbs are golden. Serve immediately, topped with chives.

TIP:
If you're in a hurry, you can skip the crispy top and oven baking, and just enjoy it as is – in which case it only takes 15 minutes.

Making it dairy-free? Or vegan?
Use the dairy-free milk of your choice and replace all of the cheese with your favourite dairy-free cheese. I'd recommend one with as much flavour as possible and, ideally, one that melts well.

ONE-PAN
Cajun 'Dirty' Rice

use a low FODMAP stock cube and omit the celery

SERVES · 3

TAKES · 20 MINUTES

- 2 tbsp garlic-infused oil
- 120g / 4¼oz smoked streaky bacon, diced
- 500g / 18oz minced (ground) beef
- 1 red (bell) pepper, diced
- 1 carrot, diced
- 1 celery stick, diced
- 250ml / 1 cup gluten-free beef stock
- 200g / generous 1 cup long-grain rice, cooked and ideally chilled
- Handful of spring onion (scallion) greens, chopped

For the Cajun spice blend
- 1 tsp smoked paprika
- ½ tsp dried chilli flakes, plus extra (optional), to serve
- ½ tsp ground cumin
- ½ tsp dried oregano
- ¼ tsp ground coriander
- Pinch of cayenne pepper
- Pinch of ground allspice
- Pinch of ground ginger

This Cajun-style fried rice is packed with tons of smoky flavour and a mildly spicy kick. The rice soaks up all that wonderful flavour from the stock, beef and veg which gives it loads of flavour and that signature 'dirty' look.

Mix together all the ingredients for your spice blend in a small bowl.

Add your garlic-infused oil to a large pan over a medium heat. Once heated, add your bacon and fry for 2–3 minutes until the fat starts to brown a little, then add your beef and fry for 2–3 minutes until browned.

Throw in your red pepper, carrot and celery and stir-fry for 3–4 minutes. Add in your spice blend and mix thoroughly until everything is well coated. Fry for a further minute until the spices become fragrant.

Next, pour in your stock and simmer for 5 minutes or until the vegetables are a little more softened. Then add in your cooked rice and stir so that it becomes really well coated in all the stock and seasoning. Keep stir-frying until the rice becomes a little more crisp and dry, instead of still being moist from the stock.

Lastly, add your spring onion greens and stir once more. Serve with extra dried chilli flakes on top, if you like a little more spice.

Making it veggie? Or vegan?
Replace the minced beef and bacon with a 400g / 14oz can of chickpeas (garbanzo beans), drained, adding them with the rice. Use a gluten-free vegetable/vegan stock cube instead of beef stock.

Mark's Mum's
MALAYSIAN CHICKEN CURRY

lactose free

dairy free

SERVES · 2–3

TAKES · 45 MINUTES

- 2 tbsp garlic-infused oil
- 500g / 18oz chicken thighs, bone in, skin on
- 2 potatoes, peeled and chopped
- 1 carrot, chopped
- 1 x 400g / 14oz can coconut milk
- 200ml / generous ¾ cup water
- 1 lemongrass stalk
- 10 dried curry leaves
- Handful of spring onion (scallion) greens, chopped, to serve

For the curry paste

- 2 tbsp mild curry powder
- 1 tbsp gluten-free soy sauce
- 1 tbsp smoked paprika
- 1 tsp dried chilli flakes
- 2 tsp minced ginger paste

Mark adapted his mum's Malaysian chicken curry recipe so that I could enjoy it and I'm so glad he did! It's creamy, mildly spicy and the chicken is so tender that it just falls off the bone. Chicken on the bone is such great value, it adds so much flavour and this is an amazing one-pot way of using it.

Mix all the curry paste ingredients in a small bowl until combined.

Grab a Dutch oven or a lidded flameproof casserole dish and place over a low heat. Add the garlic-infused oil and, once heated, add the curry paste and stir for 2 minutes until fragrant.

Add your chicken thighs and mix until well coated in the curry paste and oil, then add in your chopped potatoes and carrot, followed by the coconut milk and water. Give it a good stir until well combined, then add in your lemongrass and curry leaves. Bring to the boil, reduce the heat and allow to simmer for 30–40 minutes.

Turn off the heat and allow to cool for 5 minutes. The curry will thicken a little more as it cools. Serve with sticky jasmine rice and sprinkled with spring onion greens.

TIP:
Don't forget to remove/avoid the lemongrass stalk and curry leaves when serving!

Making it veggie? Or vegan?
Omit the chicken and continue with the recipe as directed, adding a can of drained chickpeas (garbanzo beans) 5 minutes before the curry has finished simmering.

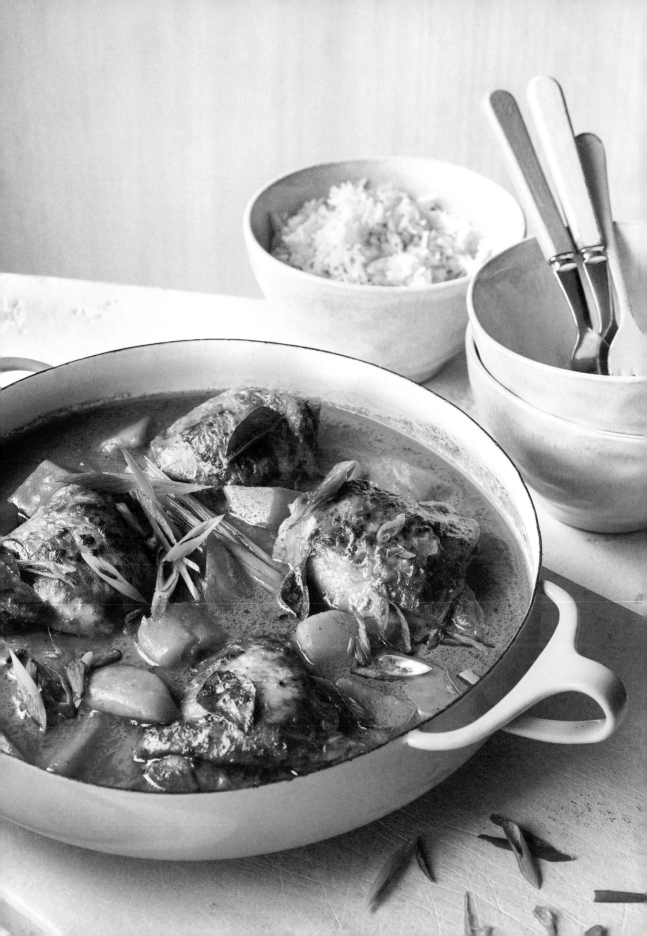

MARK'S
· Bang-Bang ·
CHICKEN STIR-FRY

swap green pepper for red instead

SERVES · 2

TAKES · 20 MINUTES

- 250g / 9oz chicken breast fillets
- 200g / 7oz dried ribbon rice noodles
- 2 tbsp garlic-infused oil
- 2 carrots, thinly sliced
- 1 green (bell) pepper, chopped
- Handful of beansprouts
- 2 handfuls of spring onion (scallion) greens, chopped
- Salt

For the sauce

- 4 tbsp gluten-free soy sauce
- 2 tbsp crunchy peanut butter
- 2 tbsp garlic-infused oil
- 2 tbsp rice wine vinegar
- 1 tbsp maple syrup
- 1 tsp dried chilli flakes
- 1 tsp minced ginger paste

To serve (optional)

- Handful of crushed roasted peanuts (ensure gluten-free)
- 2 eggs, fried

This stir-fry is the king of all stir-fries in our house. The bang-bang sauce is sweet, sour, nutty, savoury and mildly spicy all at the same time. The shredded chicken is so incredibly tender and I love the fried egg Mark always puts on top! For a little more spice, sprinkle an extra ½ tsp dried chilli flakes on top before serving.

Half-fill a small saucepan with water, add a pinch of salt and bring to the boil. Add your whole chicken fillets and bring down to a simmer. Cover and poach gently for 15 minutes until tender and cooked.

Next, add all the sauce ingredients to a small bowl. Mix until well combined and all the peanut butter is incorporated into the mixture.

Prepare your dried rice noodles according to the packet instructions (Mark places his into a mixing bowl, adds boiling water from the kettle and covers with a plate for 5 minutes). Drain and set aside.

Grab a wok, add the garlic-infused oil and place over a high heat. Add your carrots and green pepper and stir-fry until lightly browned and softened. Turn down to a medium heat, add your drained noodles and stir-fry so that they get coated in the oil and the veg is nicely mixed into them. If you're using vermicelli rice noodles instead of ribbon, don't stir too much as they break very easily - it's best to toss the mixture in the wok instead.

Remove your poached chicken from the water and place on a plate or chopping board. Using two forks, shred the chicken and throw it straight into the wok.

Next, add your sauce and stir-fry until the chicken is mixed in and everything is coated in the sauce. Lastly, add your beansprouts and spring onion greens, then stir once more until everything is mixed in. Remove from the heat and allow to sit for a minute so the beansprouts soften a little. Serve with crushed roasted peanuts and a fried egg on top, if you like.

TIP:
I find that rice noodles that also have a little tapioca starch in them are the best, as they don't break as easily as vermicelli.

Making this veggie? Or vegan?
Make this into a bang-bang cauliflower stir-fry by replacing the chicken with cooked cauliflower. Skip the egg if you're vegan.

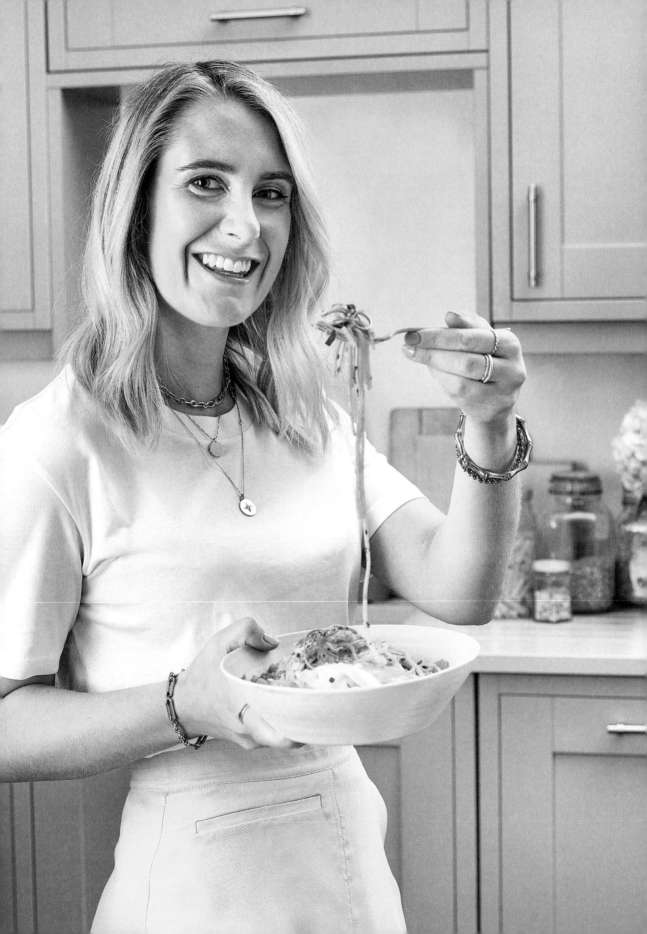

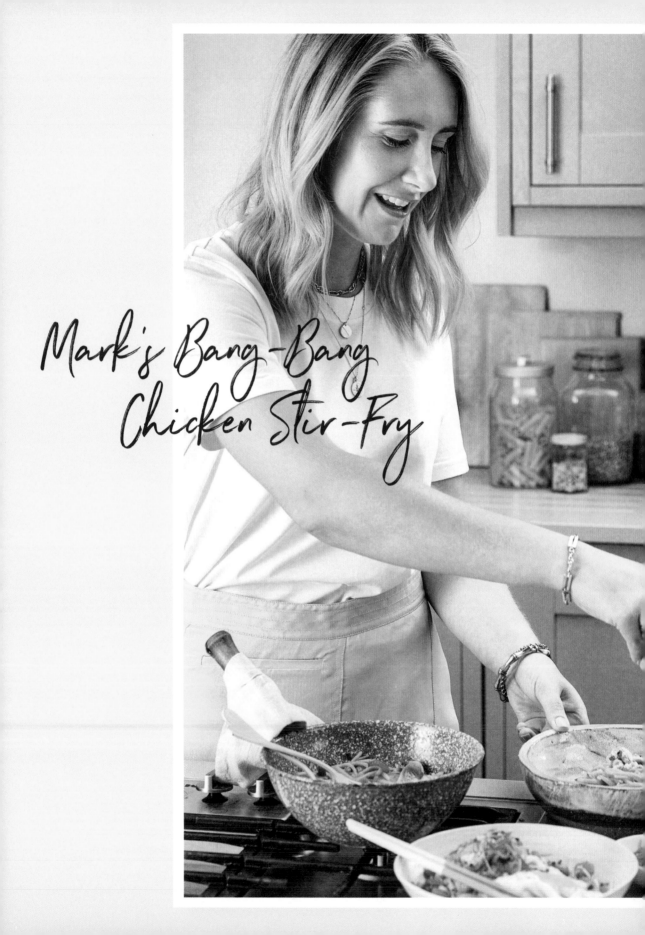

Mark's Bang-Bang
Chicken Stir-Fry

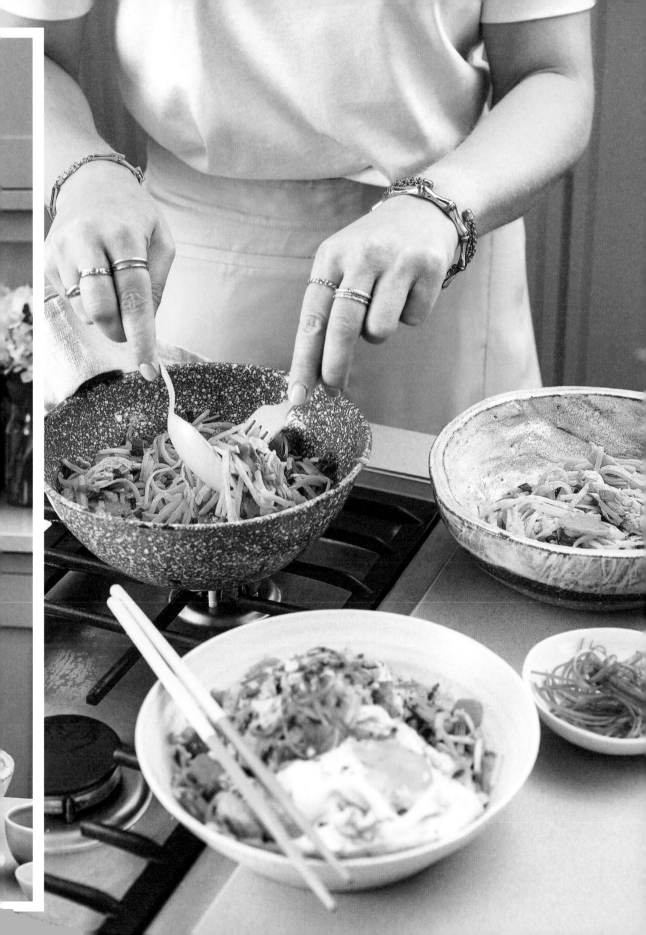

Baking

You only need to walk into any bakery on Earth to realize the true extent of how little there is in there that we can eat. And you'd definitely be forgiven for thinking that none of it could ever even be made gluten-free at home.

But since visiting some truly mind-blowing 100% gluten-free bakeries on my travels, one bite (or several thousand) made me realize that nothing is impossible. And a gluten-free 'version' certainly doesn't need to taste or look worse at all. Nobody ever even notices or cares that all my bakes are gluten-free and that's the best compliment I could possibly receive on my baking!

So this chapter is dedicated to all the baking classics that'll make you say 'I can't believe this is gluten-free.'

PS: I can't emphasize how important it is to weigh out your ingredients with digital cooking scales for gluten-free baking. The difference of 10 grams or millilitres can make a huge difference!

FRIED
Jam Doughnuts

use dairy-free milk and butter alternative

use lactose-free milk

MAKES · 12

TAKES · 30 MINUTES + 1 HOUR CHILLING

- 175g / 1⅓ cups gluten-free self-raising (self-rising) flour
- 55g / ½ cup cornflour (cornstarch)
- 60g / 5 tbsp caster (superfine) sugar
- 1 tsp gluten-free baking powder
- ¼ tsp salt
- 1 large egg
- 150ml / ⅝ cup milk
- 35g / 2½ tbsp butter, melted and cooled
- Vegetable oil, for frying

To finish

- 50g / ¼ cup caster (superfine) or granulated sugar
- Raspberry jam (jelly)

Why on Earth is it so hard to find a gluten-free jam doughnut? Well, the search is finally over. These little golden nuggets of joy are crisp on the outside, fluffy in the middle and oozing with raspberry jam. They're a little like a cross between a seaside doughnut and a filled jam doughnut - the best of both worlds!

In a large mixing bowl, add all your dry ingredients and mix until well combined. Add in the egg, milk and melted butter. Mix everything together until smooth and combined (I use an electric hand whisk for this).

Place some non-stick baking parchment on a baking tray that will comfortably fit into your freezer. Spoon your batter into a piping bag and cut off the end so that you have a nice, wide opening. Pipe your batter straight onto the non-stick baking parchment to create round discs that are 7cm / 2¾in in diameter and just over 1cm / ½in tall. If you don't have a piping bag you can carefully spoon it onto the baking parchment.

Place the baking tray in the freezer for about 1 hour. Don't skip this step! It will mean you can easily transfer the doughnut batter to the hot oil without it losing its doughnut shape.

Half-fill a large, heavy-based saucepan with vegetable oil and place it over a medium heat for 15 minutes or until the oil reaches 170°C / 340°F - test the temperature of the oil with a cooking thermometer or by using the wooden spoon handle test (page 19).

Remove the chilled doughnut discs from the freezer. Carefully remove them from the baking parchment and gently lower them, in batches, into your hot oil. Cook for 6–8 minutes, turning occasionally.

The doughnuts will initially sink but will then come up to the surface of the oil and start to float. Once nice and golden on both sides, remove from the oil using a slotted spoon, place on some kitchen paper and allow to drain.

When cool enough to handle, spread your sugar onto a large plate. Toss your doughnuts in the sugar until well coated.

To fill the doughnuts, place your jam in a piping bag with a small nozzle, ideally a long filling nozzle. Use a chopstick or a skewer to make a hole in the side of each doughnut. Push the nozzle into the hole and generously pipe the jam into the middle - the more the better!

Enjoy the doughnuts straight away while they're still warm, or later at room temperature - or simply reheat them in the microwave.

TIPS:
You can happily leave the doughnut shapes on a tray in the freezer for as long as you like. Then simply continue the recipe from the point of frying whenever you fancy some! Feel free to pipe the batter into rings before freezing to make fried ring doughnuts.

Making it vegan?
Use dairy-free milk and a vegan alternative to butter. Replace the egg with 3 tbsp aquafaba (whisked until frothy).

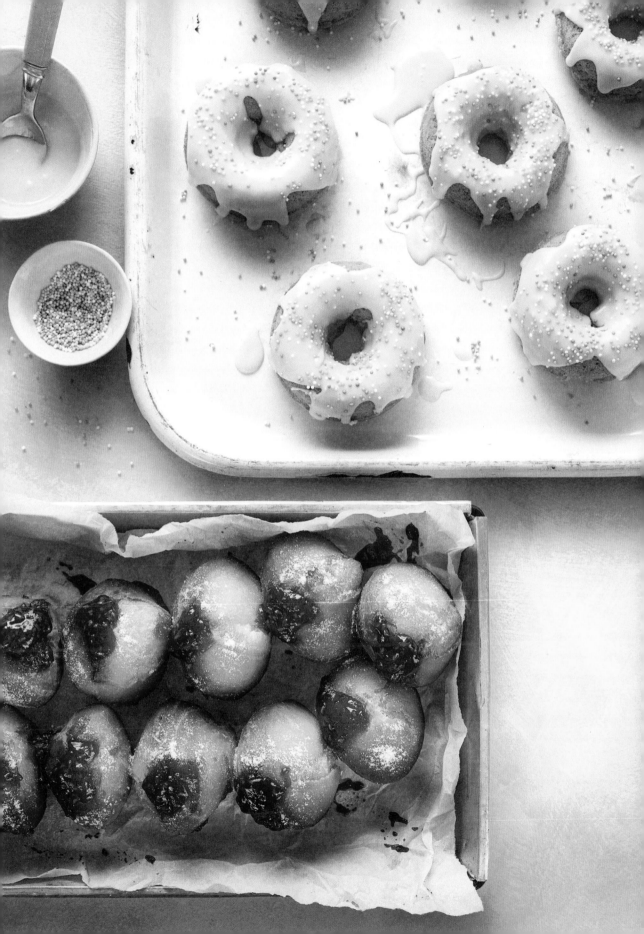

BAKED RING
Doughnuts

 use dairy-free milk and a hard dairy-free butter alternative

 use lactose-free milk

 use lactose-free milk

MAKES · 15

TAKES · 45 MINUTES

- Butter or oil, for greasing

For the doughnuts

- 150ml / ⅝ cup milk
- 1 tbsp lemon juice
- 345g / 2⅔ cups gluten-free self-raising (self-rising) flour
- 175g / ¾ cup plus 3 tbsp caster (superfine) sugar
- ¼ tsp xanthan gum
- 1 tsp ground cinnamon (optional)
- 75g / ⅓ cup butter, melted and cooled
- 50g / 1¾oz vegetable oil
- 2 large eggs
- 1 tsp vanilla extract

For the sugar coating

- 75g / ⅓ cup butter, melted
- 150g / ¾ cup granulated sugar

OR

For the icing

- 85g / generous ½ cup icing (confectioners') sugar
- 3 tbsp milk
- 1 tsp vanilla extract
- Food colouring (or any colour you like)
- Multi-coloured sprinkles (ensure gluten-free)

My baked ring doughnuts are super soft and light, with two ways to finish them. You can either go for a crunchy, sugared coating, or a sweet, glazed finish with sprinkles – 'Homer Simpson' doughnuts as I call them! Looking for a fried doughnut finish? Try my jam doughnuts on page 150.

Preheat your oven to 160°C fan / 180°C / 350°F. Prepare a doughnut tin (pan) by greasing each hole with butter or a little oil.

In a jug (pitcher), mix your milk and lemon juice and leave to stand for 10 minutes until it curdles a little.

In a large mixing bowl, add your flour, sugar, xanthan gum and cinnamon and mix until well combined.

Grab another mixing bowl and add your cooled, melted butter, oil, eggs, vanilla and curdled milk mixture. Whisk until combined.

Pour your wet ingredients into your dry ingredients and mix together, whisking by hand until just combined, then immediately stop mixing. Definitely don't over-mix this one! Spoon your mixture into your prepared doughnut tin, right to the top of each hole. Bake in the oven for 15 minutes until risen and golden. Allow to cool in the tin, then carefully transfer to a wire rack.

It's totally up to you how you finish them! For a simple sugar finish, roll the doughnuts in a bowl of melted butter while still warm, then roll on a large plate of sugar until well coated.

For a glazed ring doughnut finish, wait until the doughnuts have fully cooled. Grab a mixing bowl and add your icing sugar, milk and vanilla. Mix until it reaches a smooth, slightly thick but pourable consistency. Add a tiny amount of the food colouring, stirring it in and adding a few drops at a time until you achieve your desired colour. I always seem to go for bright pink doughnuts!

Dip the top of your doughnuts into the icing bowl and then cover in sprinkles. Allow to set on a wire rack.

Pictured on page 151

Making it vegan?
Use dairy-free milk and a vegan alternative to butter. Replace the eggs with 6 tbsp aquafaba (whisked until frothy). Ensure the food colouring is vegan.

Triple Chocolate
BROWNIES

use lactose-free chocolate and cocoa powder

use dairy-free chocolate, cocoa powder and a hard dairy-free butter alternative

MAKES · 9

TAKES · 45 MINUTES

- 250g / 1 cup plus 2 tbsp butter, plus extra for greasing
- 125g / 4½oz dark chocolate, broken into pieces
- 125g / 4½oz milk chocolate (or more dark chocolate), broken into pieces
- 100g / ¾ cup gluten-free plain (all-purpose) flour
- 50g / ½ cup cocoa powder
- 4 medium eggs (or 3 large eggs)
- 280g / scant 1½ cups caster (superfine) sugar
- 60g / 2oz white chocolate chips
- 60g / 2oz milk chocolate chips
- 60g / 2oz dark chocolate chips

For the last decade, the only gluten-free option on offer always seemed to be a gluten-free brownie. And the standard 'varied' to put it politely! So here's my game-changing, intensely fudgy and chocolatey gluten-free brownies that will hopefully restore your faith in them.

Preheat your oven to 160°C fan / 180°C / 350°F. Lightly grease a 23cm / 9in square baking tin (pan) and line with non-stick baking parchment.

In a large heatproof bowl, add the butter and both chocolates. Place over a saucepan of gently boiling water, making sure the water isn't touching the bowl, stirring until everything has melted and mixed together. Once melted, allow to cool to near room temperature. You can also melt your butter and chocolate in the microwave in short bursts, stirring between each burst.

Sift your flour and cocoa powder into a medium mixing bowl, then mix together.

In a large mixing bowl, whisk your eggs and sugar until lighter in colour (I use an electric hand whisk or a stand mixer for this). Pour your cooled, melted chocolate mixture into your egg and sugar mixture and carefully fold it in with a spatula until glossy and chocolatey in colour. Fold in your flour and cocoa mixture until well combined, then fold in your chocolate chips so that they're evenly distributed.

Spoon the mixture into your prepared tin, smoothing it over to create a nice, even layer. Bake in the oven for 35–40 minutes until it develops a shiny, paper-like crust on top. Allow to cool completely in the tin. Once cooled, slice and enjoy.

TIPS:
For a more cakey brownie, leave in the oven for an extra 5–10 minutes.

For an even more fudgy brownie, pop them in the fridge for an hour after they've cooled.

ONE BOWL
Choc chip
BANANA BREAD

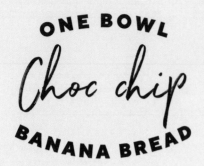

use lactose-free choc chips

use dairy-free choc chips and a dairy-free butter alternative

MAKES · 1 LOAF (12 SLICES)

TAKES · 1 HOUR 10 MINUTES

- 115g / ½ cup butter, softened, plus extra for greasing
- 115g / ½ cup plus 1 tbsp light brown sugar
- 2 medium eggs, beaten
- 500g / 18oz ripe bananas, mashed
- 250g / 1¾ cups plus 2 tbsp gluten-free plain (all-purpose) flour
- ¼ tsp xanthan gum
- 1 tsp bicarbonate of soda (baking soda)
- 1 tsp ground cinnamon
- 150g / 5¼oz chocolate chips

If humans are 60% water, then I must therefore be 40% banana bread at a minimum. When every bite is packed with tons of scrumptious banana flavour and chunky chocolate chips, it's not particularly hard to understand why, is it?

Preheat your oven to 160°C fan / 180°C / 350°F. Lightly grease a 900g / 2lb loaf tin (pan) and line with non-stick baking parchment.

In a large mixing bowl, cream together your softened butter and sugar until light and pale (I use an electric hand whisk or a stand mixer for this). Add your beaten eggs and mashed banana and mix until well combined.

Add your flour, xanthan gum, bicarb and cinnamon and mix briefly until no dry flour can be seen. Lastly, add in three-quarters of your chocolate chips and mix once more.

Spoon the mixture into your prepared tin and sprinkle the rest of your chocolate chips on top. Cook in the oven for 1 hour until golden – check that it's cooked by sticking a skewer into the centre – if it comes out clean, then it's done.

Allow to cool briefly in the tin, then carefully lift onto a wire rack. Slice and enjoy.

Making it vegan?
Add 2 more small bananas (mashed and ripe) in place of the eggs. Use dairy-free chocolate chips and a dairy-free butter alternative.

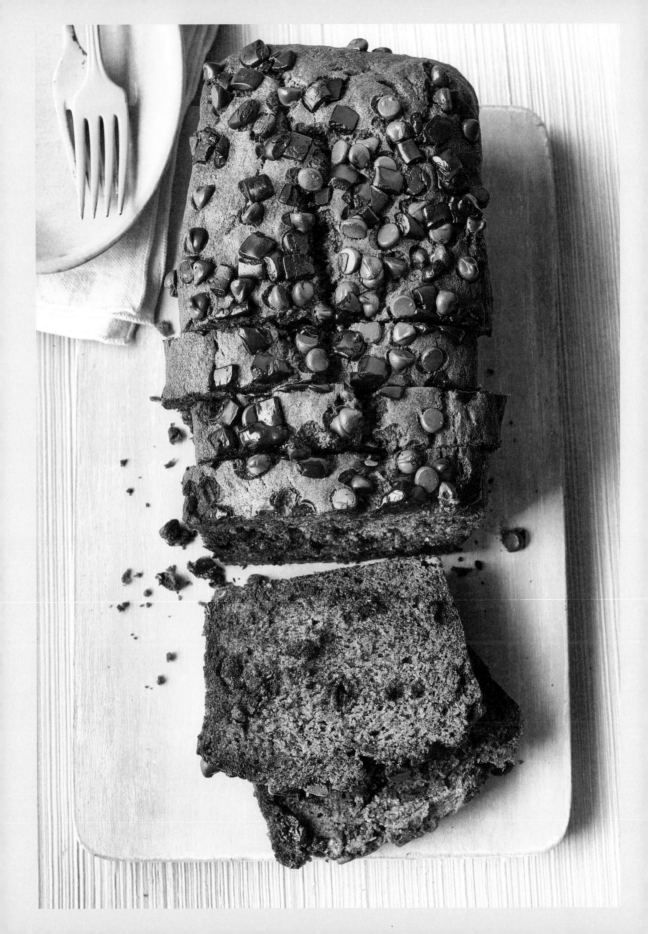

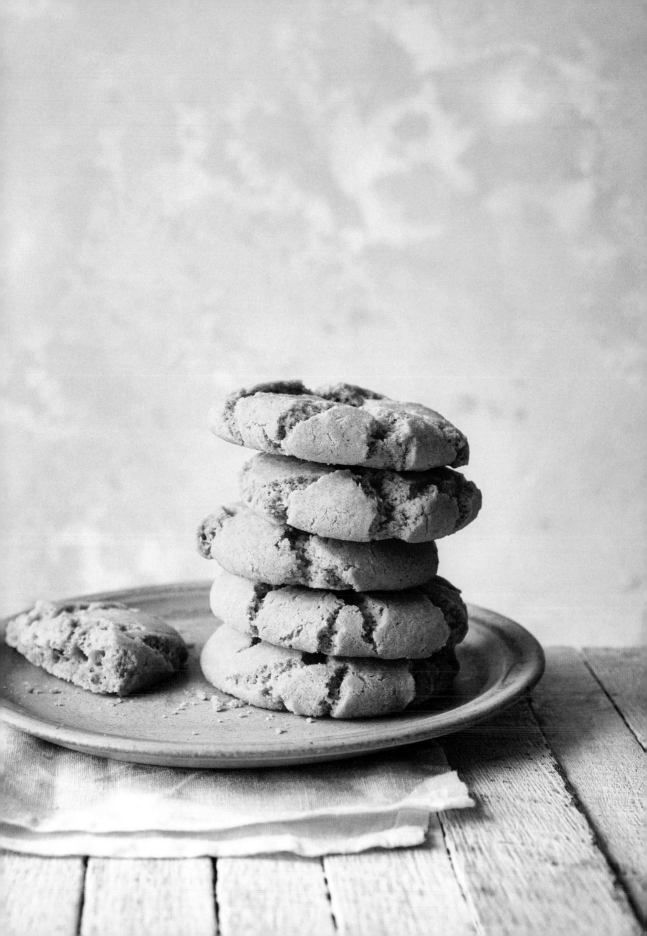

Grandma's
GINGER BISCUITS

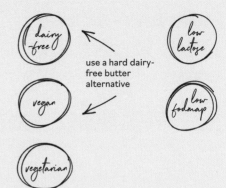

dairy-free

low lactose

vegan

use a hard dairy-free butter alternative

low fodmap

vegetarian

MAKES · 15

TAKES · 30 MINUTES

- 240g / 1¾ cups plus 1 tbsp gluten-free self-raising (self-rising) flour
- ¼ tsp xanthan gum
- 100g / ½ cup caster (superfine) sugar
- 100g / ½ cup light brown sugar
- 2 tsp ground ginger
- 85g / ⅓ cup cold butter, cubed
- 1 tbsp golden syrup
- 1 tsp bicarbonate of soda (baking soda)
- 1½ tbsp water

Nobody made ginger biscuits quite like my grandma. Of course, I adapted them to be gluten-free but I'm sure she wouldn't mind! They're crisp on the outside and chewy in the middle, with a sweet, warming hug of ginger. I'm not sure she ever thought they'd one day appear in a recipe book, but she'd be so happy that so many people now get to enjoy them – as am I!

Preheat your oven to 140°C fan / 160°C / 325°F. Line two large baking trays with non-stick baking parchment.

In a large mixing bowl, combine your flour, xanthan gum, both sugars and ginger. Add your chopped butter and rub it in with your fingers until it forms a breadcrumb-like consistency. Next, add your golden syrup then mix your bicarb and water together and add to the mixture. Mix together until it forms a dough, then use your hands to bring it together into a ball.

Roll small portions of your dough into small, even balls and place on the baking trays. I weigh each ball to ensure they're all the same size – mine were 30g / 1oz each. Leave a generous amount of room around each ball as they'll spread in the oven.

Cook in the oven for 18–20 minutes, until flattened and golden. They will be very soft at first so allow to cool on the trays before moving them to a wire rack to cool completely.

BAKERY-STYLE
Choc Chip Cookies

 use dairy-free choc chips and a hard dairy-free butter alternative

 use lactose-free choc chips

 use lactose-free choc chips

MAKES · 15

TAKES · 20 MINUTES

- 125g / ½ cup plus 1 tbsp butter, softened
- 100g / ½ cup light brown sugar
- 100g / ½ cup caster (superfine) sugar
- 1 large egg
- 1 tsp vanilla extract
- 225g / 1¾ cups gluten-free self-raising (self-rising) flour
- ½ tsp bicarbonate of soda (baking soda)
- ½ tsp salt
- 225g / 8oz chocolate chips (white, milk or dark)

These are exactly the same as those thin, bakery-style cookies that are crisp on the outside, packed with chocolate chips and chewy in the middle. The only difference is that you can actually eat these, for once! They're super quick to make as there's no need to chill them.

Preheat your oven to 180°C fan / 200°C / 400°F. Line two large baking trays with non-stick baking parchment.

In a large mixing bowl, cream together your softened butter and both sugars until light, fluffy and well combined.

Crack in the egg, add your vanilla and mix in. Next, add your flour, bicarb and salt, and mix well. Lastly, add your chocolate chips and mix in so that they're well distributed.

Roll your dough into small, even-sized balls and place on the lined baking trays. (I weigh each ball to ensure they're all the same size – mine were 40g / 1½oz each.) The dough might be a little sticky, but that's fine. Leave a generous amount of room around each ball as they'll spread in the oven.

Bake in the oven for 9–10 minutes until a tiny bit golden on all the edges. They will feel very soft to touch when they come out, so leave to cool briefly on the trays before transferring to a wire rack to cool. You can enjoy them warm or completely cooled.

TIP:
For a slightly more 'cookie dough' centre, freeze your cookie balls before baking, for 30 minutes. They won't spread as much in the oven and will be lovely and chunky in the middle. You can also roll your cookie dough into larger balls, and cook for longer, if you want bigger cookies.

Making it vegan?
Use dairy-free chocolate chips and a (hard) dairy-free alternative to butter. Replace the egg with 3 tbsp aquafaba (whisked until frothy).

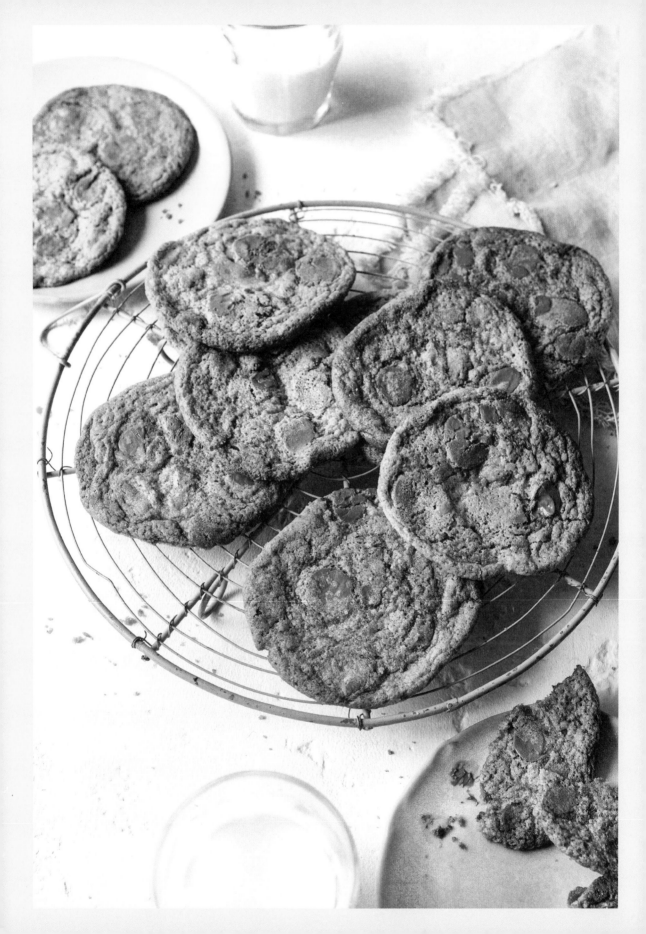

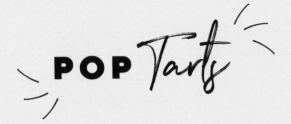

POP Tarts

low lactose — use lactose-free milk

low fodmap — use lactose-free milk

dairy free — use dairy-free milk

vegetarian

MAKES · 5

TAKES · 45 MINUTES

- 1 quantity of gluten-free shortcrust pastry (page 27), chilled for 25 minutes
- Gluten-free plain (all-purpose) flour, for dusting
- 1 egg, beaten with 2 tsp milk

For the jam filling

- 150g / ½ cup raspberry jam (jelly)
- 1 tbsp cornflour (cornstarch)
- 1 tsp lemon juice

For the icing

- 200g / 1½ cups icing (confectioners') sugar
- 1 tsp vanilla extract
- Multi-coloured sprinkles (ensure gluten-free)

It's been over a decade since I last ate a pop tart, how about you? Thankfully, making your own is incredibly simple and fun – perfect if you have little helpers in the kitchen too. Plus, they taste a million miles better than a regular pop tart! However, I wouldn't recommend toasting them once cooled as the icing will melt!

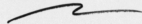

Preheat your oven to 160°C fan / 180°C / 350°F. Line a large baking tray with non-stick baking parchment.

In a small bowl, mix the jam, cornflour and lemon juice until well combined. Set aside.

Remove your pastry from the fridge – if your dough feels really firm when you take it out, leave it out at room temperature briefly before rolling it. Don't handle your dough excessively as this will warm it up and make it more fragile.

Lightly flour your rolling pin. On a sheet of non-stick baking parchment, roll out the dough to a rectangle, 2mm / 1⁄16in thick. Cut as many 10 x 7.5cm / 4 x 3in rectangles out of your pastry as you can. Use a palette knife to gently place them to one side while you reroll your pastry scraps to cut out more rectangles.

Brush around the border of half of your rectangles with some of your beaten egg mixture, then add a tablespoon of your jam

mixture and spread, leaving a 1.5cm / ½in clear border around the edge. Using a fork, prick some holes in the remaining rectangles (which will allow steam to escape when baking).

Place these rectangle lids on top of the ones with jam on and gently press the edges down so they stick together. Then, using a fork, press down on the edges all the way around to crimp together. Transfer to the baking tray, brush the top of each pop tart with a little more beaten egg and bake in the oven for 20–22 minutes until golden. Remove from the oven and carefully transfer to a wire rack and allow to fully cool.

For the icing, grab a medium-sized mixing bowl and add your icing sugar and vanilla. Mix together, gradually adding a few teaspoons of water and mixing until it reaches a smooth, slightly thick and spreadable consistency. If your icing is too thin, it'll dribble off the pop tart!

Once the pop tarts have fully cooled, spoon a dollop of the icing onto the centre of each and neatly spread up to the crimped edge. Add a few sprinkles and repeat until you've decorated all of your pop tarts. Allow to set and enjoy.

TIP:
If you don't have time to make your own pastry, use store-bought gluten-free pastry instead.

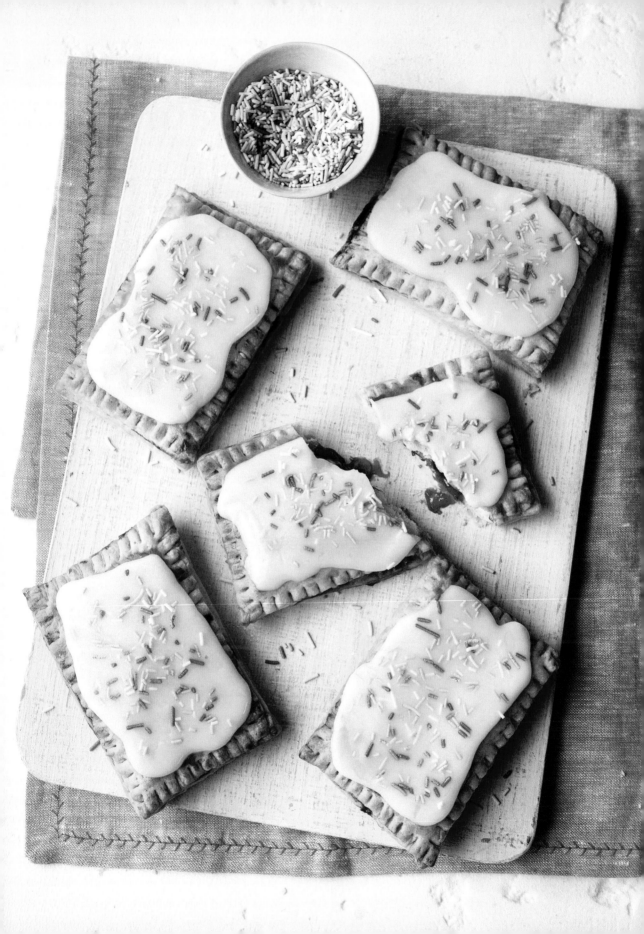

.ONE-BOWL.
Blueberry Muffins

 use dairy-free milk

 use lactose-free milk

 use lactose-free milk

MAKES · 15

TAKES · 30 MINUTES

- 180ml / ¾ cup milk
- 1 tbsp lemon juice
- 130ml / ½ cup plus 1 tbsp vegetable oil
- 1 large egg
- Grated zest of 1 lemon
- 200g / 1 cup caster (superfine) sugar
- 1 tsp bicarbonate of soda (baking soda)
- ¼ tsp xanthan gum
- 300g / 2¼ cups gluten-free self-raising (self-rising) flour, plus 1 tsp for the blueberries
- 200g / 1½ cups fresh blueberries
- 4 tbsp demerara sugar

These light and fluffy muffins are packed with bursting blueberries, finished with a shimmering, crunchy, sugared top. This recipe is incredibly versatile so if you want to replace the blueberries with chocolate chips, then go for it! Just skip adding the lemon if so.

Preheat your oven to 160°C fan / 180°C / 350°F. Line a 12-hole muffin tray with muffin or tulip cases. In a jug (pitcher), mix your milk and lemon juice and allow to stand for 10 minutes until it curdles a little.

In a large mixing bowl, add your oil, milk mixture, egg and lemon zest. Mix until combined and smooth, using a hand whisk. Next, add in your caster sugar, bicarb, xanthan gum and flour. Whisk by hand until just combined then immediately stop mixing. Be gentle and don't over-whisk!

Mix the berries with the teaspoon of flour to stop them from sinking in the batter. Then carefully fold your blueberries into the batter. Spoon your mixture into the muffin cases, dividing it evenly.

Sprinkle 1 teaspoon of demerara sugar on top of each muffin, then bake in the oven for 22–25 minutes until golden. Check they're cooked by sticking a skewer into the centre of a muffin – if it comes out clean, then they're done. Bear in mind that you might hit a gooey blueberry!

Allow to cool in the muffin tray, then carefully transfer your muffins to a wire rack to cool.

Making it vegan?
Use dairy-free milk. Replace the egg with 3 tbsp aquafaba (whisked until frothy).

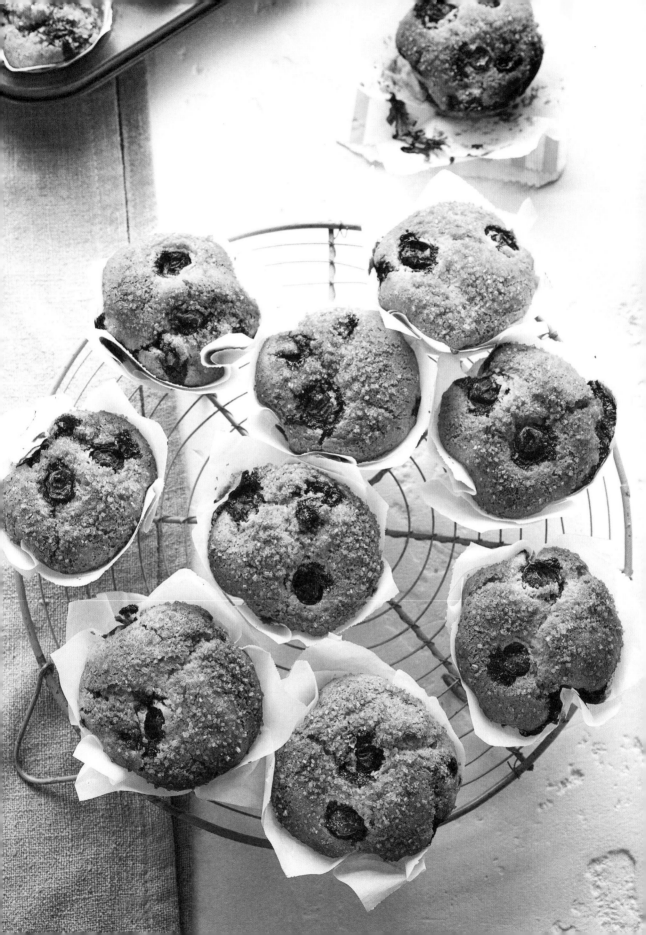

White Chocolate &
RASPBERRY CUPCAKES

 use dairy-free white chocolate and a hard dairy-free butter alternative

 use lactose-free white chocolate

 use lactose-free white chocolate

MAKES · 12

TAKES · 35 MINUTES

- 175g / ¾ cup plus 3 tbsp caster (superfine) sugar
- 175g / ¾ cup plus 1 tsp butter, softened
- 170g / 1⅓ cups gluten-free self-raising (self-rising) flour
- 3 large eggs, beaten
- ½ tsp vanilla extract
- ½ tsp gluten-free baking powder
- ¼ tsp xanthan gum
- 125g / 1 cup fresh raspberries, plus extra (optional) to decorate
- 100g / 3½oz white chocolate chips

For the buttercream

- 125g / 4½oz white chocolate, plus extra (optional) to decorate
- 150g / ⅔ cup butter, softened
- 300g / 2 cups icing (confectioners') sugar

White chocolate and raspberry is one of my favourite flavour combos when it comes to baking. With soft vanilla cupcakes packed with white choc chips, fresh raspberries and tons of fluffy white chocolate icing, you absolutely can't go wrong.

Preheat your oven to 160°C fan / 180°C / 350°F. Line a 12-hole cupcake tray with cupcake cases. I like to sprinkle a few grains of dried rice beneath each case as it helps to absorb unwanted moisture.

In a large mixing bowl, cream together your sugar and butter until light and pale (I use an electric hand whisk or a stand mixer for this). Add your flour, beaten eggs, vanilla, baking powder and xanthan gum. Mix until well combined. Carefully fold in your fresh raspberries and white chocolate chips.

Spoon your mixture evenly into the cupcake cases and bake in the oven for 20–25 minutes until golden. Check that they're cooked by sticking a skewer into the centre of a cupcake – if it comes out clean, then they're done. Bear in mind that you might hit a gooey raspberry!

Allow to cool in the cupcake tray then carefully transfer to a wire rack to cool completely.

To make your buttercream, melt your chocolate either in the microwave (in short bursts, stirring in between) or in a heatproof bowl set over a pan of boiling water, making sure the base of the bowl isn't touching the water. Allow to cool.

Mix your butter in a stand mixer on a medium speed for 5 minutes or until pale. Add your icing sugar in three stages and beat for about 3 minutes between each addition. Start your mixer slowly to save your kitchen from an icing sugar explosion, but make sure you remember to increase the speed back to medium for each of your 3-minute mixing intervals.

Once your icing sugar is fully mixed in, add your cooled, melted chocolate. Beat for 2–3 more minutes until well combined, and the buttercream is smooth, light and fluffy.

(You can of course make the buttercream using an electric hand whisk too. Also, while making the buttercream by hand requires a little extra time and elbow grease, it's more than possible! I'd recommend sifting your icing sugar first if making it by hand.)

You can then either use a piping bag with an open star nozzle to pipe the icing on, or simply spoon the buttercream onto the cooled cupcakes. Optionally add some grated white chocolate and a fresh raspberry to each as a finishing touch.

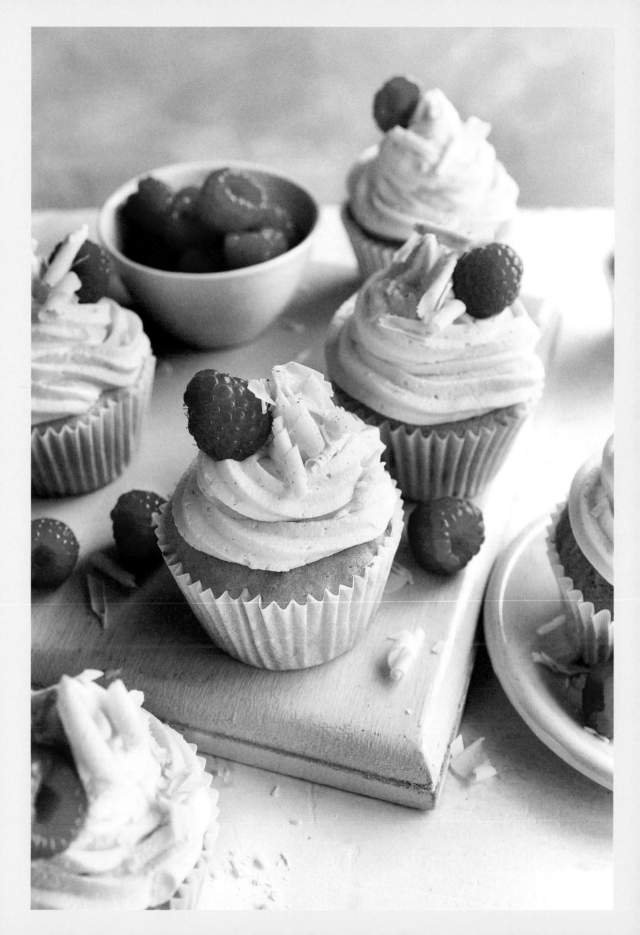

. Ultimate .
CHOCOLATE
FUDGE CAKE

use lactose-free milk, chocolate, cream and cocoa powder

MAKES · 1 CAKE (12 SLICES)

TAKES · 1 HOUR

- Butter, for greasing
- 190ml / generous ¾ cup milk
- 1 tbsp lemon juice
- 200g / 1½ cups gluten-free plain (all-purpose) flour
- 50g / ½ cup cocoa powder
- 160g / ¾ cup plus 1 tbsp caster (superfine) sugar
- 150g / ¾ cup light brown sugar
- 1 tsp gluten-free baking powder
- 1 tsp bicarbonate of soda (baking soda)
- ½ tsp xanthan gum
- 2 medium eggs
- 80ml / ⅓ cup melted butter (or oil), cooled
- 1 tbsp vanilla extract
- 1 tbsp instant coffee
- 190ml / ¾ cup plus 1 tbsp boiling water

For the icing

- 200g / 7oz dark chocolate, broken into pieces
- 155g / ⅔ cup butter
- 90ml / 6 tbsp double (heavy) cream

When a chocolate cake isn't chocolatey enough, make my chocolate fudge cake. The cake itself is incredibly fudgy with a rich, deep chocolate flavour and the icing is indulgently creamy. Combine the two and you've basically got every chocaholic's dream! The coffee brings out the deep chocolate flavour, so don't worry – it doesn't taste like coffee at all.

Preheat your oven to 160°C fan / 180°C / 350°F. Lightly grease two 20cm / 8in round cake tins (pans) and line with non-stick baking parchment.

Start by making your icing. In a large heatproof bowl, add your chocolate, butter and cream. Place over a saucepan of gently boiling water, making sure the water isn't touching the base of the bowl, and keep stirring until everything has melted and mixed together. Set aside to cool completely and thicken to a spreadable consistency.

In a medium-sized mixing bowl, mix your milk and lemon juice and allow to stand for 10 minutes until it curdles a little.

In a large mixing bowl, add all the dry ingredients, sifting in the flour and cocoa powder. Mix well.

Crack your eggs into the slightly curdled milk, then add the melted butter or oil, and vanilla. Beat until smooth. Add the wet mixture to your dry ingredients and mix together until well combined.

Next, dissolve the coffee in the boiling water and add to the cake mixture. Mix until it has a nice shine to it, then split your mixture evenly between the two tins.

Bake for 30–35 minutes, checking that the cakes are cooked by sticking a skewer into the centre – if it comes out clean, then they're done. Leave to cool for 10 minutes in the tins before turning out onto a wire rack to cool completely.

Spoon the icing onto one of the cooled cakes and spread evenly to the edges. Place your other cake on top, spoon more icing on top and evenly spread it to the edges, adding enough for the icing to just start going over the edges – you can then spread the icing around the sides too so that the cake is completely covered.

Slice and enjoy!

Making it dairy-free?
Replace the butter with a (hard) dairy-free alternative to butter. Ensure the chocolate and cocoa powder are both dairy-free. Use dairy-free milk. Use a dairy-free alternative to double cream.

Making it vegan?
Follow the advice above to make it dairy-free, and replace the eggs with 6 tbsp aquafaba (whisked until frothy).

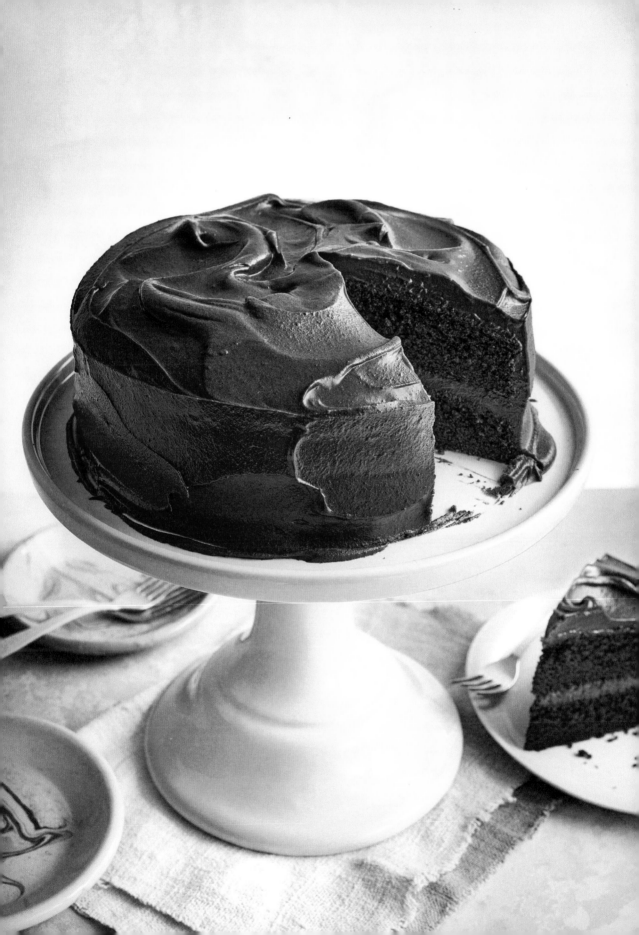

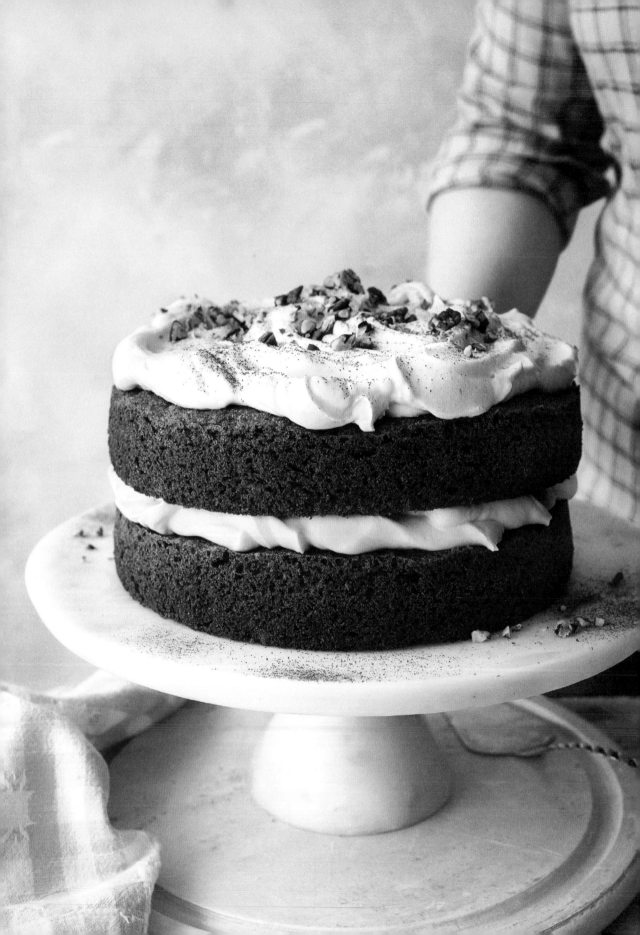

CLASSIC
Carrot Cake

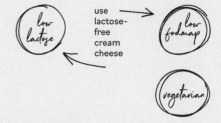

low lactose → use lactose-free cream cheese → low fodmap

vegetarian

MAKES · 1 CAKE (12 SLICES)

TAKES · 45 MINUTES

- Butter, for greasing
- 4 eggs
- 190g / scant 1 cup light brown sugar
- 40g / 3 tbsp caster (superfine) sugar
- 200ml / generous ¾ cup vegetable oil
- 265g / 2 cups gluten-free self-raising (self-rising) flour
- 1½ tsp bicarbonate of soda (baking soda)
- 2 tsp ground cinnamon
- 1 tsp ground ginger
- Grated zest of 1 large orange
- 250g / 9oz carrots, grated
- 60g / ⅔ cup pecans, finely chopped (optional)

For the cream cheese icing
- 150g / ⅔ cup butter, softened
- 150g / 1 cup icing (confectioners') sugar
- 300g / 1⅓ cups cream cheese (must be full-fat)
- 1 tsp vanilla extract

To finish (optional)
- Dusting of ground cinnamon
- Handful of pecans, finely chopped

I've never met anyone who a) didn't like this cake or b) even noticed that it was gluten-free. It's incredibly soft and moist, with a subtle yet warming hint of cinnamon and ginger. The fluffy cream cheese frosting is the icing on the cake... quite literally!

Preheat your oven to 160°C fan / 180°C / 350°F. Lightly grease two 20cm / 8in round cake tins (pans) and line with non-stick baking parchment.

In a large mixing bowl, crack in your eggs, then add both sugars and your oil. Mix together until well combined (I use an electric hand whisk or a stand mixer for this).

In a separate bowl, sift in your flour, bicarb, cinnamon and ginger. Add this dry mixture to the wet mixture and gently fold in. Add your orange zest, grated carrots and chopped pecans, if using. Fold into the mixture so that the carrots and orange zest are evenly dispersed.

Split your mixture evenly between the two tins and bake in the oven for 30 minutes until golden. Check that the cakes are cooked by sticking a skewer into the centre of a cake – if it comes out clean, then it's done. Allow to cool in the tins, then carefully transfer to a wire rack.

To make your cream cheese icing, mix your softened butter in a stand mixer on a medium speed for 5 minutes or until pale. Add your icing sugar in two stages and beat for about 3 minutes between each

addition. Start your mixer slowly to save your kitchen from an icing sugar explosion but make sure you remember to increase the speed back to medium for each of your 3-minute mixing intervals.

Add in your cream cheese and vanilla and beat for 2–3 more minutes until well combined, and the icing is light and fluffy, without lumps.

(You can make the cream cheese icing using an electric hand whisk too. Also, while making the icing by hand requires a little extra time and elbow grease, it's more than possible! I'd recommend sifting your icing sugar first if making it by hand.)

Once cooled, spoon the icing onto one of the cakes and spread evenly to the edges. Place your second cake on top and spoon more icing on top, evenly spreading it to the edges. Dust with a little extra cinnamon and top with chopped pecans, if you like.

TIP:
As this cake uses cream cheese icing, it must be stored in the fridge in an airtight container.

Making it dairy-free?
Replace the butter with a (hard) dairy-free alternative to butter for the icing. Also use a dairy-free alternative to cream cheese and gradually add a little extra icing sugar until the icing comes together. I also recommend chilling the cream cheese frosting when making dairy-free if it seems a bit looser.

COFFEE AND
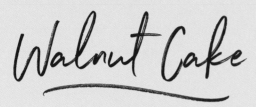
Walnut Cake

 low lactose

 low fodmap

 vegetarian

**MAKES · 1 CAKE
(12–16 PIECES)**

TAKES · 1 HOUR

- 350g / 1½ cups butter, softened, plus extra for greasing
- 350g / 1¾ cups light brown sugar
- 6 eggs
- 350g / 2⅔ cups gluten-free self-raising (self-rising) flour
- ¼ tsp xanthan gum
- 4 tsp instant coffee, mixed with 1½ tbsp boiling water and cooled
- 100g / 1 cup walnuts, finely chopped or blitzed into small chunks in a food processor

For the coffee buttercream

- 200g / scant 1 cup butter, softened
- 420g / 3 cups icing (confectioners') sugar
- 4 tsp instant coffee, mixed with 1½ tbsp boiling water and cooled

To finish

- 50g / ½ cup walnuts, roughly chopped

My coffee and walnut traybake (sheet cake) has that undeniable, deep, rich coffee flavour that's softened with sweet, caramel notes from the light brown sugar. Each bite is full of added crunch thanks to the chopped walnuts, and who could forget that sweet, coffee-infused icing? A definite hit with coffee lovers and coffee dodgers alike!

Preheat your oven to 160°C fan / 180°C / 350°F. Lightly grease a 33 x 23cm / 13 x 9in rectangular baking tin (pan) and line with non-stick baking parchment.

In a large mixing bowl, cream together your softened butter and sugar until light and pale (I use an electric hand whisk or a stand mixer for this).

Gradually add your eggs, one at a time, mixing in between each addition. Fold the flour and xanthan gum into the mixture, pour in your cooled coffee mixture and fold in once again. Add your finely chopped walnuts and carefully fold in.

Spoon the mixture into the prepared baking tin and bake in the oven for 45 minutes until cooked – check by sticking a skewer into the centre: if it comes out clean, then it's done. Allow to cool in the tin then carefully transfer to a wire rack to cool completely.

To make your coffee buttercream, mix your softened butter in a stand mixer on a medium speed for 5 minutes or until pale. Add your icing sugar in two stages and beat for about 3 minutes between each addition – start your mixer slowly to save your kitchen from an icing sugar explosion, but make sure you remember to increase the speed back to medium for each of your 3-minute mixing intervals.

Next, gradually add your cooled coffee mixture. Beat for 2–3 more minutes until well combined, light and fluffy.

(You can make the buttercream using an electric hand whisk. Also, while making the buttercream by hand requires a little extra time and elbow grease, it's more than possible! I'd recommend sifting your icing sugar first if making it by hand.)

Finally, spread the coffee buttercream all over the top of your now fully cooled cake. Cut into squares, then finish by decorating the top with chopped walnuts.

TIP:

If you want to make this into a round cake instead of a traybake (sheet cake), reduce the flour, sugar and butter to 225g (1¾ cups, generous 1 cup and 1 cup respectively), reduce the eggs to 4, and reduce the walnuts to 70g / ¾ cup. Bake in two 20cm / 8in round tins for 25 minutes at the same temperature.

Making it dairy-free?
Replace the butter with a (hard) dairy-free alternative to butter. You might also need to add a little extra icing sugar when making the buttercream until it comes together.

Swiss ROLL

use dairy-free milk and make buttercream using a hard dairy-free butter alternative

use lactose-free milk and fill with buttercream

SERVES · 6

TAKES · 25 MINUTES

- 2 tbsp vegetable oil, plus extra for greasing
- 4 medium eggs, separated
- 100g / ½ cup caster (superfine) sugar
- ½ tsp vanilla extract
- 2 tbsp milk
- 60g / ½ cup minus 1 tbsp gluten-free plain (all-purpose) flour
- ¼ tsp xanthan gum
- 1 tbsp icing (confectioners') sugar or caster sugar
- 4 tbsp jam (jelly)

For a fresh cream filling

- 200ml / generous ¾ cup double (heavy) cream
- 1 tbsp icing (confectioners') sugar

OR

For a buttercream filling

- 100g / scant ½ cup butter, softened
- 200g / 1½ cups icing (confectioners') sugar
- ½ tsp vanilla extract

A Swiss roll was something that I always believed was impossible to make gluten-free. How could you possibly roll a gluten-free sponge without it breaking into a million crumbs?! Well, with this recipe, you can! With an incredibly light and fluffy sponge, smothered in jam and the choice of a cream or buttercream swirl, one slice is never enough.

Preheat your oven to 180°C fan / 200°C / 400°F. Lightly grease a Swiss roll tin (pan) and line with non-stick baking parchment.

In a large mixing bowl, add your egg yolks and half the caster sugar. Whisk together until combined, then add your vanilla, milk and oil and whisk once more. Sift in the flour and add the xanthan gum, and mix in until well combined, thick and glossy.

In a separate bowl, whisk your egg whites, using an electric hand whisk or stand mixer, until they start to turn white and frothy. You can do this by hand, but be prepared to spend extra time reaching that frothy point. Gradually add the remaining caster sugar, whisking until you have medium peaks.

In a few stages, add your egg white mixture to your egg yolk mixture, folding it in carefully between each addition. Once all the egg white mixture is fully folded in, pour your mixture into your prepared tin. Spread it out gently to make sure it's nice and even and bake in the oven for 10–12 minutes until golden.

Place a piece of non-stick baking parchment on your work surface and dust it with the icing or caster sugar.

While your sponge is still warm, loosen it from the tin and flip it out onto the parchment. Peel off the parchment that lined the tin – don't worry if you lose the outer layer of the cake that sticks to the paper as you peel it off, that's totally normal. Using your baking parchment, roll the sponge up from the short

end – the parchment should be inside it as you roll. Try to roll fairly tightly, then leave the sponge to fully cool while rolled up.

While the sponge is cooling you can prepare the filling. It's totally up to you how to finish them!

For a fresh cream filling, whip your cream with the icing sugar until thick and stiff.

For a buttercream filling, mix your softened butter in a stand mixer on a medium speed for 5 minutes or until pale. Add your icing sugar in two stages and beat for about 3 minutes between each addition. Start your mixer slowly to save your kitchen from an icing sugar explosion, but make sure you remember to increase the speed back to medium for each of your 3-minute mixing intervals. Next, gradually add your vanilla. Beat for 2–3 more minutes until well combined and the buttercream is light and fluffy.

Once the sponge is cool, carefully unroll it and spread your jam followed by your chosen cream filling over it; don't put too much on or go too close to the edges, or it will spill out.

Reroll up the sponge without the parchment inside this time. Dust with a little extra sugar. Allow to briefly chill in the fridge before slicing up and serving.

TIP:

It's vital to roll the sponge up using parchment while it's still warm from the oven. If you allow it to cool and then try to roll it up, I guarantee you that it will break and crack horrendously!

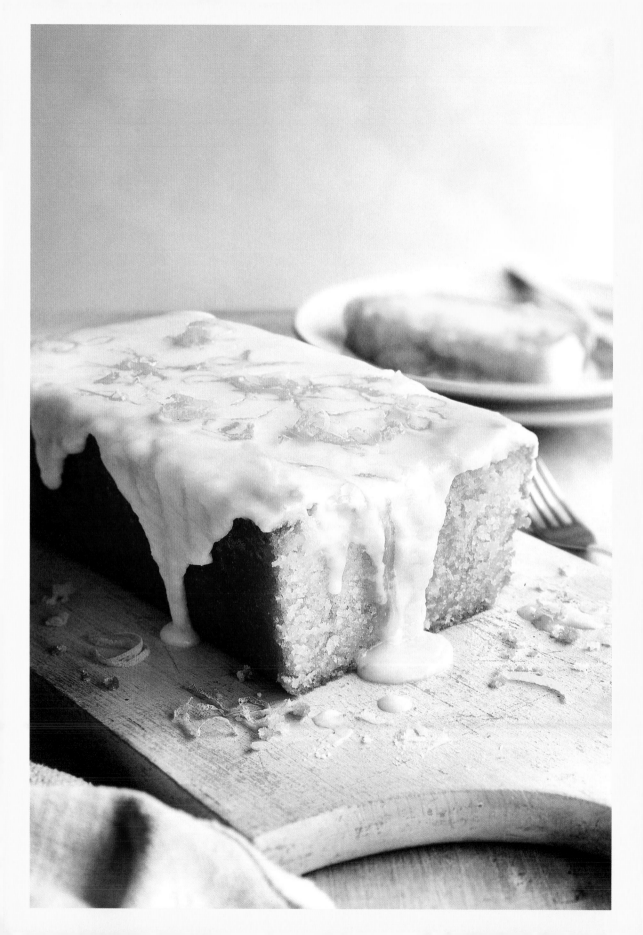

Lemon Drizzle CAKE

use a dairy-free butter alternative

MAKES · 12 SLICES

TAKES · 1 HOUR 15 MINUTES

- 175g / ¾ cup plus 1 tsp butter, softened, plus extra for greasing
- 175g / ¾ cup plus 3 tbsp caster (superfine) sugar
- Grated zest of 2 lemons
- 3 medium eggs
- 100g / ¾ cup gluten-free self-raising (self-rising) flour
- 75g / ¾ cup ground almonds

For the drizzle

- 100g / ½ cup caster (superfine) sugar
- Grated zest of 1 lemon and juice of 2 (juice the ones you used in the cake)

For the icing

- 120g / generous ¾ cup icing (confectioners') sugar
- Grated zest of 1 lemon and juice of 2

This has been a favourite on the blog for years, so I absolutely had to include it in my first ever recipe book. It's incredibly soft thanks to the drizzle, packed with lemon flavour and topped with a zesty, lemon-infused icing. My secret ingredient is ground almonds – it makes the cake so lovely and moist!

Preheat your oven to 160°C fan / 180°C / 350°F. Lightly grease a 900g / 2lb loaf tin (pan) and line with non-stick baking parchment.

In a large mixing bowl, cream together your softened butter and sugar until light and pale (I use an electric hand whisk or a stand mixer for this). Add the lemon zest and beat once more until light and fluffy. Crack in the eggs, one at a time, mixing in between until well combined. Sift in your flour and fold it in, then fold in your ground almonds.

Spoon the mixture into your prepared tin and bake in the oven for 45–50 minutes until golden. If it's browning too much on top, cover with foil (shiny side up) for the final 5–10 minutes.

While the cake is baking, make the drizzle. Grab a small mixing bowl, add the sugar, lemon zest and juice, and mix until well combined.

Remove your cake from the oven. Check that it's cooked by sticking a skewer into the centre – if it comes out clean, then it's done. Use a skewer to poke lots of holes all over the top of the cake, while it's still hot. Then gradually pour over all of the drizzle. Allow to cool briefly in the tin then carefully lift onto a wire rack to cool completely.

For the icing, grab a medium bowl and add your icing sugar and lemon juice. Mix until it reaches a smooth, slightly thick, yet still pourable consistency. Once the cake has fully cooled, drizzle the icing all over the top of the cake and sprinkle with the lemon zest.

MALT *loaf*

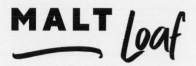

vegetarian

dairy free

lactose free

use oil for greasing

MAKES · 1 LOAF (12 SLICES)

TAKES · 2 HOURS 20 MINUTES

- Butter or oil, for greasing
- 300ml / 1¼ cups strong tea (made with 3 tea bags)
- 150g / 1 cup mixed dried fruit, such as raisins and sultanas (golden raisins)
- 200g / 1 cup dark brown sugar
- 1 tbsp black treacle (molasses)
- 1 large egg, beaten
- 270g / 2 cups gluten-free self-raising (self-rising) flour
- ½ tsp xanthan gum
- 1 tsp ground mixed spice
- 2 tbsp golden syrup (optional)

Say hello to my own gluten-free version of the classic malt loaf – with no gluten-y malt in sight. Each slice is packed with raisins and has a lovely, chewy texture, with a deep, warming sweetness thanks to the black treacle. Simply slice, spread with butter and enjoy.

Place your strong tea and mixed dried fruit into a large bowl. Allow it to sit for no less than 1 hour.

Preheat your oven to 160°C fan / 180°C / 350°F. Lightly grease a 900g / 2lb loaf tin (pan) and line with non-stick baking parchment.

Next, add your sugar, treacle, beaten egg, flour, xanthan gum and mixed spice. Mix together until thoroughly combined.

Spoon your mixture into your lined tin and bake in the oven for 1 hour 20 minutes until golden on top. Remove from the oven and check that it's cooked by sticking a skewer into the centre - if it comes out clean, then it's done.

Allow to cool briefly in the tin, topping with golden syrup, if you like, while still warm. Leave to cool completely on a wire rack, before slicing and enjoying spread with butter or a dairy-free alternative.

Making it vegan?
Replace the egg with 3 tbsp aquafaba (whisked until frothy). Use oil for greasing instead of butter.

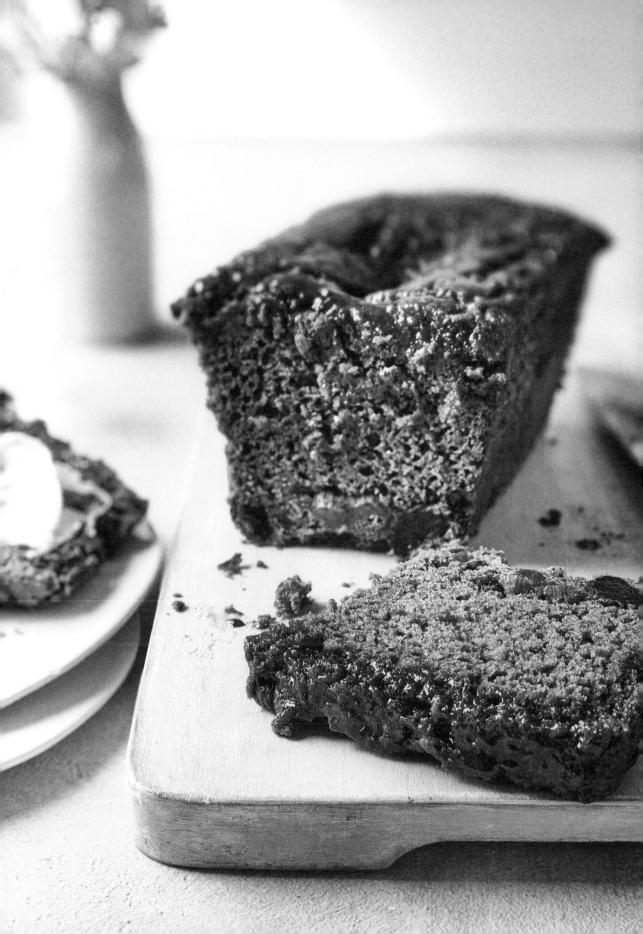

VANILLA, LEMON OR CHOCOLATE
· Birthday Cake ·

**MAKES · 1 CAKE
(12 PIECES)**

**TAKES · 45 MINUTES
PLUS COOLING AND ICING**

For the sponge cake base

- 225g / 1 cup butter, softened, plus extra for greasing
- 225g / 1 cup plus 2 tbsp caster (superfine) sugar
- 4 eggs
- 225g / 1¾ cups gluten-free self-raising (self-rising) flour
- 1 tsp gluten-free baking powder
- ¼ tsp xanthan gum

For a vanilla sponge

- 1 tsp vanilla extract
- Raspberry or strawberry jam (jelly)
- Multi-coloured sprinkles (ensure gluten-free)

For a lemon sponge

- Grated zest of 4 lemons, plus 1 tsp juice
- Lemon curd

For a chocolate sponge

- 40g / 6 tbsp cocoa powder (reduce flour to 185g / 1¼ cups)
- Chocolate sprinkles (ensure gluten-free)

For the buttercream icing (frosting) base

- 375g / 1⅔ cups butter, softened
- 750g / generous 5 cups icing (confectioners') sugar

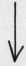

For vanilla icing (frosting)

- 1½ tsp vanilla extract

For lemon icing (frosting)

- Grated zest of 3 lemons
- 3 tbsp lemon juice

For chocolate icing (frosting)

- 90g / scant 1 cup cocoa powder, sifted, or 225g / 8oz dark chocolate, melted and cooled

This recipe is fully customizable in three ways, to make either a vanilla, lemon or chocolate cake. It uses the all-in-one method for the sponge which makes this so quick and easy to prepare. Best of all, nobody would ever even know this is gluten-free, so everyone can enjoy it together. Consider this recipe your birthday present from me (no, you can't have the receipt).

Preheat your oven to 160°C fan / 180°C / 350°F. Lightly grease the bases of two 20cm / 8in round cake tins (pans) and line with non-stick baking parchment.

In a large mixing bowl, add all the ingredients for your sponge base. **If making a vanilla sponge**, add your vanilla. **If making a lemon sponge**, add the zest of 3 lemons (saving the zest of 1 lemon for decorating) and the juice. **If making a chocolate sponge**, remember to reduce the flour and sift in the cocoa powder instead.

Mix until well combined for around 1 minute (I use an electric hand whisk or a stand mixer for this).

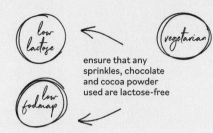

low lactose

vegetarian

ensure that any sprinkles, chocolate and cocoa powder used are lactose-free

low fodmap

Split your mixture evenly between the two tins and bake in the oven for 25–30 minutes until cooked – check by sticking a skewer into the centre of a cake: if it comes out clean, then it's done. Allow to cool in the tins then carefully lift onto a wire rack to fully cool.

To make your buttercream icing, place your softened butter in a stand mixer and mix on a medium speed for 5 minutes or until the butter has turned pale. Add your icing sugar in three stages and beat for about 3 minutes between each addition. Start your mixer slowly to save your kitchen from an icing sugar explosion, but make sure you remember to increase the speed back to medium for each of your 3-minute mixing intervals.

If making vanilla icing, add your vanilla. **If making lemon icing**, add your lemon zest and juice. **If making chocolate icing**, add either your sifted cocoa powder or melted chocolate.

Beat for 2–3 more minutes until well combined, smooth, light and fluffy.

(You can of course make the buttercream using an electric hand whisk too. Also, while making the buttercream by hand requires a little extra time and elbow grease, it's more than possible! I'd recommend sifting your icing sugar first if making it by hand.)

Once your sponges have fully cooled, you can now ice and construct your cake.

For a vanilla cake, spoon jam onto one of the sponges and spread evenly to the edges. On the underside of the second sponge, spread a layer of your vanilla buttercream evenly to the edges. Place your second cake on top, buttercream-side down. Continue to cover the top and sides of your cake with the rest of the buttercream. Top with sprinkles, pop in some candles and serve.

For a lemon cake, do the same as above, but spread the lemon curd on the first sponge in place of jam and use your lemon buttercream to ice. Sprinkle your reserved lemon zest over the top, pop in some candles and serve.

For a chocolate cake, spoon a layer of your chocolate icing onto one of the sponges and spread evenly to the edges. Place your other cake on top. Continue to cover the top and sides of your cake with the rest of the buttercream. Top with your chocolate sprinkles, pop in some candles and serve.

TIPS:
For a three-tiered birthday cake with added wow-factor, simply make an extra sponge, more buttercream and increase the vanilla / lemon / chocolate additions. Do this by multiplying all measurements by 1.5. It's best to write down the new measurements to avoid confusion!

You can also finish your cakes with fondant icing on top instead of buttercream, if you fancy. These sponges are strong enough to hold that type of icing just fine!

Want to make your own lemon curd? There's a simple lemon curd recipe over on my blog, which you can use.

Pictured on pages 178–9

Making it dairy-free?
Use a (hard) dairy-free alternative to butter and ensure everything used is dairy-free, like the lemon curd, cocoa powder and melted chocolate, if using. You'll also need to gradually add a little extra icing sugar when making the buttercream until it comes together. I recommend chilling the buttercream when making dairy-free if it seems a bit loose.

Vanilla Birthday Cake

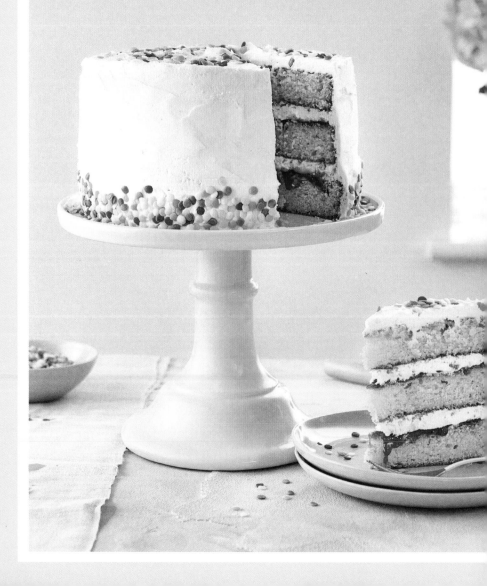

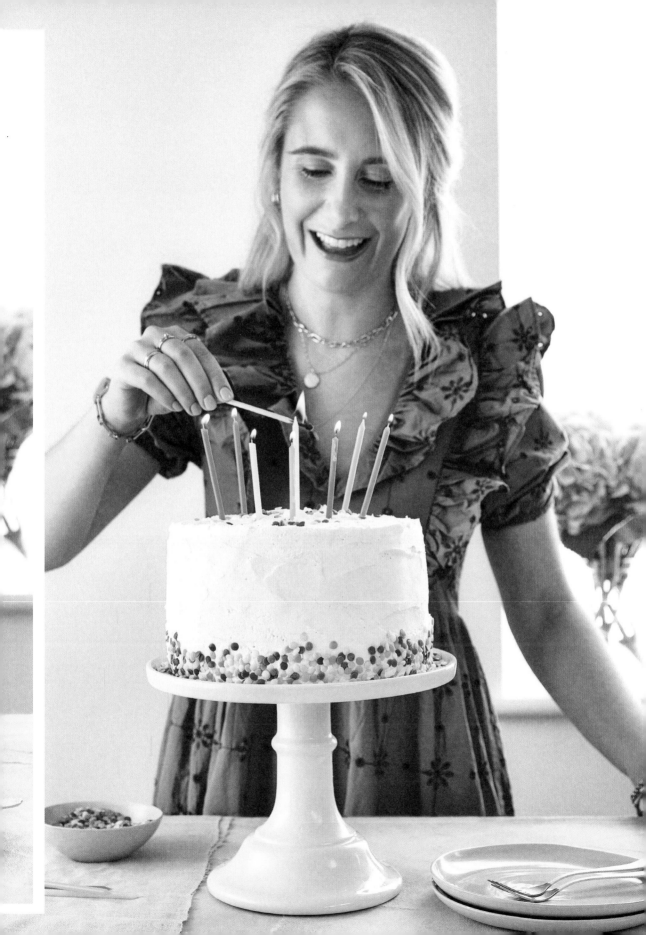

Bakewell TART

use a hard dairy-free butter alternative

use 15g / ½oz flaked almonds

MAKES · 12 SLICES

TAKES · 1 HOUR

- 1 quantity of gluten-free shortcrust pastry (page 27), chilled for 25 minutes
- 4 tbsp raspberry jam (jelly)
- Handful of flaked (slivered) almonds

For the frangipane

- 125g / ½ cup plus 1 tbsp butter, softened
- 125g / ⅔ cup caster (superfine) sugar
- 2 eggs, beaten
- 125g / 1¼ cups ground almonds
- 1 tsp almond extract
- 25g / 3 tbsp gluten-free plain (all-purpose) flour
- ½ tsp gluten-free baking powder

This classic British tart is a symphony of buttery pastry, sweet raspberry jam and a lovely, light almond frangipane. I first made this in food tech at school and I've understandably lost count of how many times I've made it since – obviously, it's gluten-free now!

Remove your pastry from the fridge. If it feels really firm when you take it out, leave it out at room temperature briefly before rolling it. Don't handle it excessively as this will warm it up and make it more fragile.

Lightly flour your rolling pin. On a sheet of non-stick baking parchment, roll out the pastry to a large circle 3mm / ⅛in thick. Transfer to a 23cm / 9in fluted tart tin (pan), by supporting the pastry as you gently invert it into the tin, with equal overhang on all sides. Peel off the baking parchment.

Next, use your fingers to carefully ease the pastry into place so that it neatly lines the tin. Lift the overhanging pastry and, using your thumb, squash 2mm / ¹⁄₁₆in of pastry back into the tin. This will result in slightly thicker sides, which will prevent your pastry case from shrinking when baked. Allow the overhang to do its thing – we'll trim the overhang after chilling it.

Lightly prick the base of the pastry case with a fork then place in the fridge for 15 minutes. Preheat the oven to 180°C fan / 200°C / 400°F and place a baking tray inside to heat up.

After chilling, use a rolling pin to roll over the top of the tin, neatly removing the overhang and flattening down the pastry. Loosely line the base of the pastry case with baking parchment and fill with baking beans (or uncooked rice if you don't have any). Bake in the oven on the heated tray for 15 minutes, then remove the parchment paper and beans and bake for a further 5 minutes. Remove from the oven and allow to fully cool. Reduce the oven temperature to 160°C fan / 180°C / 350°F.

Next, prepare your frangipane. In a large mixing bowl, cream together your softened butter and sugar until light and pale (I prefer to do this using an electric hand whisk). Gradually add in your beaten eggs and mix again until combined. Fold in your ground almonds, almond extract, flour and baking powder.

Spread your raspberry jam onto the base of your cooled pastry case and spoon your frangipane mixture on top of the jam, spreading it out so it's nice and level, ideally using a palette knife. Sprinkle with your flaked almonds.

Bake in the oven for 35–40 minutes until golden and the top is no longer wobbly. Remove from the oven and allow to cool completely in the tin. Serve warm or cold.

TIPS:

You can also add glacé icing on top of your Bakewell tart once it has cooled. Just mix together 275g / scant 2 cups icing (confectioners') sugar with 1 tsp almond extract and enough water to get to the right consistency. Drizzle it messily over the top or cover the whole thing in one smooth layer. Allow it to fully set before slicing.

If you don't have time to make your own pastry, use store-bought gluten-free pastry instead.

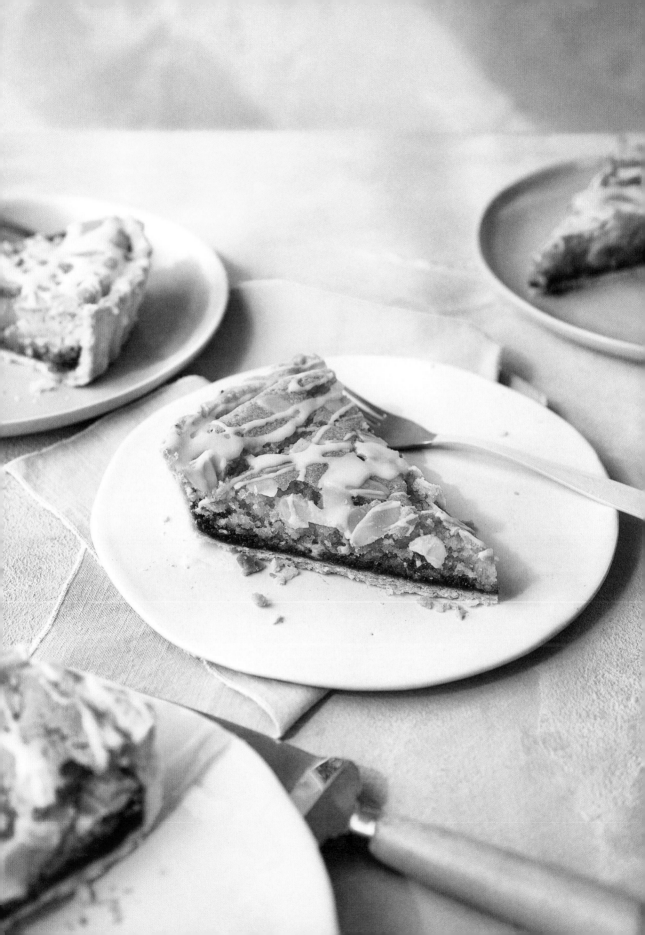

Pastéis de Nata

(PORTUGUESE CUSTARD TARTS)

use dairy-free milk for custard and oil for greasing

 use lactose-free milk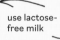

MAKES · 12

TAKES · 50 MINUTES

- Butter or oil, for greasing
- 1 quantity of gluten-free rough puff pastry (page 28)
- 40g / 4¾ tbsp gluten-free plain (all-purpose) flour, plus extra for dusting
- 150ml / 10 tbsp milk
- ½ tsp vanilla extract
- 120g / ½ cup plus 1½ tbsp caster (superfine) sugar
- 1 cinnamon stick
- 80ml / ⅓ cup water
- 3 egg yolks

I quickly learned that holding my breath and waiting for a gluten-free pastéis de nata to exist wasn't a great strategy. But using my homemade gluten-free rough puff pastry and a simple 6-ingredient filling, I can now breathe a sigh of relief! That light, buttery, flaky pastry filled with creamy custard was definitely well worth the 10-year wait.

Lightly grease a 12-hole muffin tray with butter or a little oil.

Divide the pastry in half, then on a lightly floured surface, roll out one half into a long rectangle, about 30 x 15cm / 12 x 6in. Repeat with your second pastry half. Tightly roll up each pastry half from a short side, so that they form a log shape, then cut each into 6 equal rounds.

Place each round into a hole in your muffin tray. Keeping your fingers cold and slightly wet, push down with your thumb to form a well. Carefully push the pastry up the edges so that it forms a mini pastry case. Do this carefully, always pushing up from the bottom of the muffin hole. Place your muffin tray in the fridge to keep cool.

To make your custard filling, place your flour and 50ml / 3½ tbsp of the milk in a large mixing bowl and whisk together until smooth. In a small saucepan, heat up the rest of your milk until just boiling. Remove from the heat and pour into the mixing bowl. Add your vanilla and whisk until combined.

Add the sugar, cinnamon stick and water to a (clean) saucepan and mix before placing over the heat, then don't mix it again. Heat slowly until just over 100°C / 210°F. If you don't have a cooking thermometer, simply bring the mixture to boiling point, then remove from the heat.

Remove the cinnamon stick and add the hot syrup to your milk and flour mixture, whisking constantly. Once it's all incorporated, continue to whisk for about 5 minutes, until the mixture is slightly cooler. Add the egg yolks and whisk once more to combine. You can use the mixture straight away or leave it to fully cool and use later.

Preheat your oven to 240°C fan / 260°C / 500°F (or as hot as your oven will go if it doesn't reach these temperatures).

Pour your custard mixture into the pastry cases, leaving just under a 1cm / ½in gap at the top of each. Bake in the oven for about 15 minutes until the pastry is golden and the custard is nicely coloured.

Allow to cool slightly in the tray then carefully transfer your tarts to a wire rack. Enjoy slightly warm, or allow to fully cool.

TIPS:
Remember that when using rough puff pastry, you cannot simply just reroll it (or any off-cuts) into a ball. You'll destroy the layers you've spent time creating! If you do have any off-cuts, you can always bake them and roll them in cinnamon sugar for a sweet, buttery treat.

If you don't have time to make your own pastry, use store-bought gluten-free pastry instead.

Pictured on page 184

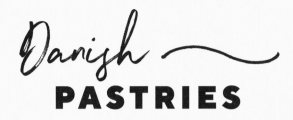

Danish
PASTRIES

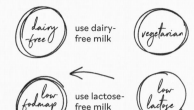

dairy-free — use dairy-free milk

vegetarian

low fodmap — use lactose-free milk

low lactose

MAKES · 8-10

**TAKES · 45 MINUTES
+ AT LEAST 2 HOURS
CHILLING**

- 1 quantity of gluten-free rough puff pastry (page 28)
- Gluten-free plain (all-purpose) flour, for dusting
- 1 egg, beaten
- Raspberry or strawberry jam (jelly), optional
- Pecans, hazelnuts or flaked (slivered) almonds, chopped (optional)
- 150g / 1 cup icing (confectioners') sugar
- 2 tsp water

For the crème pâtissière filling

- 450ml / generous 1¾ cups whole milk
- 2 tsp vanilla extract
- 150g / ¾ cup caster (superfine) sugar
- 40g / 2 tbsp cornflour (cornstarch)
- 2 eggs, plus 2 egg yolks

Gluten-free Danish pastries have always been in the top 5 on my bucket list. And once I nailed gluten-free rough puff pastry, I immediately made these. Every bite is packed with buttery, flaky, puffy pastry and a creamy custard, chopped nuts and a sweet icing. They were every bit as good as I remembered! Feel free to experiment with different fillings too.

Start by making the crème pâtissière. In a large saucepan, heat the milk and vanilla extract over a medium heat until just before it begins to boil.

In a large mixing bowl, add the sugar, cornflour, eggs and egg yolks and whisk until well combined and slightly paler.

Gradually pour the hot milk into the egg mixture, whisking in between each addition. Keep whisking continuously until it's all combined. Pour the mixture back into your saucepan and place over a medium heat. Whisk for around 5 minutes until it thickens, then continue whisking for 2 minutes. Remove from the heat and transfer to a clean bowl. If you notice any lumps in your custard in the pan – don't worry! You can always sieve it into the clean bowl.

Cover the top with cling film (plastic wrap) so the cling film is touching the surface of the custard (this will prevent a skin from forming as it cools). Place in the fridge for 2–3 hours to completely cool and further thicken.

Preheat your oven to 200°C fan / 220°C / 425°F. Line a baking tray with non-stick baking parchment.

Roll out the pastry out on a well floured surface to a rectangle 2mm / ⅟₁₆in thick. Keep flouring the surface if it gets sticky – this often happens on warmer days or if you have warm hands! Cut your pastry into 10cm / 4in squares.

Dab a little beaten egg in the centre of each square then fold each corner of the pastry inwards towards the centre so that they meet in the middle. Press down so they hold together. Place each pastry square on the baking tray and brush each with beaten egg. Spoon 1 tablespoon of crème pâtissière onto the centre of each, plus a dollop of jam and a sprinkling of chopped nuts, if you like.

Bake in the oven for 15–20 minutes until golden, then remove and leave to cool.

To finish, mix together your icing sugar with the water until it reaches a thick yet pourable consistency, then drizzle some over the top.

TIPS:
Remember that when using rough puff pastry, you cannot simply just reroll it (or any off-cuts) into a ball. You'll destroy the layers you've spent time creating! If you do have any off-cuts, you can always brush them with egg, spoon on a little pastry cream, bake and enjoy.

If you don't have time to make your own pastry, use store-bought gluten-free pastry instead.

Any extra crème pâtissière filling can be kept in the fridge for a few days and used in lots of different desserts, such as my caramel profiteroles and chocolate éclairs (pages 202 and 204).

Pictured on page 184

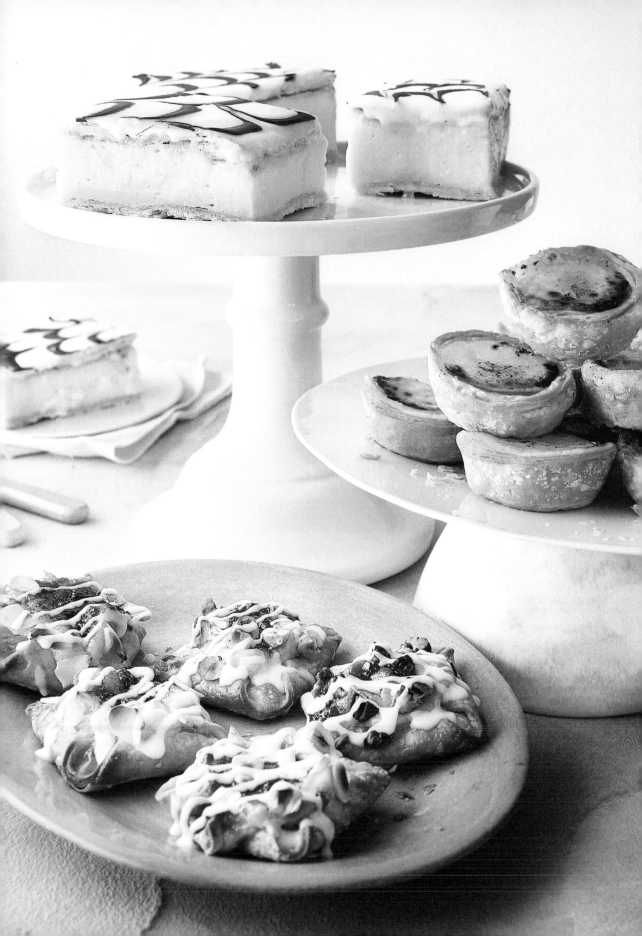

Custard
SLICE

 use dairy-free milk and chocolate

 use lactose-free milk and dairy-free chocolate

MAKES · 6

**TAKES · 1 HOUR
+ 6 HOURS CHILLING**

- 1 quantity of gluten-free rough puff pastry (page 28)

For the filling
- 1l / 4 cups milk
- 2 tsp vanilla extract
- 120g / 1¾ cups cornflour (cornstarch)
- 200g / 1 cup caster (superfine) sugar
- 4 eggs

For the icing
- 50g / 1¾ oz dark chocolate, melted
- 100g / scant ¾ cup icing (confectioners') sugar
- About 2 tbsp water

Here's another classic that tons of you guys said you'd eat first, if you could miraculously eat gluten again for one day. With a super thick layer of set custard between two sheets of golden pastry, topped with sweet icing, this is a reunion that was well worth waiting for.

Preheat your oven to 180°C fan / 200°C / 400°F. Line a baking tray with non-stick baking parchment.

Place the pastry on a large sheet of baking parchment, cut in half and roll the first portion into a large square, around 21cm / 8in and 2mm / ⅛in thick. Repeat for the other half of the dough.

Transfer the two pastry squares to the lined tray, using the parchment to lift them. Place another piece of parchment on top of the pastry then place a heavy baking tray on top of that (this will stop the pastry from rising in the oven). Bake in the oven for 15–20 minutes until golden (lift the top tray up a little to check). Remove from the oven and transfer the squares to a wire rack to cool.

To make your custard filling, heat your milk and vanilla in a saucepan over a medium heat until just boiling. In a large bowl, add your cornflour, sugar and eggs. Mix until pale and smooth.

Ladle a small amount of the hot milk into the egg mixture and mix together until fully combined, then pour the contents of the bowl into your saucepan. Place back over a low–medium heat and keep mixing. Once it starts to simmer, continue to simmer for 3 minutes until really nice and thick. Keep stirring all the time.

Remove the custard from the heat and continue to stir for a few minutes to help it cool down. Transfer to a clean bowl to help it cool further – you want it to be slightly warm but not piping hot.

Line the base and sides of a 23cm / 9in square baking tin (pan) with foil. Leave a little foil overhanging so you can easily lift out the custard slices once set. Place one pastry square in the bottom of the tin. Cut the other pastry square into 6 rectangles, each about 11 x 7cm / 4½ x 2¾in.

Once the custard has cooled until just warm, spoon it on top of the bottom pastry sheet in the baking tin, smoothing it over with a palette knife so it's an even layer. Place your rectangles of pastry on top of the custard, leaving no gaps. It doesn't matter if you don't have complete coverage around the outside edge of the tin and some custard is still visible. Place in the fridge to chill while you make your icing.

Transfer your melted chocolate to a piping bag fitted with a small, round nozzle. In a large mixing bowl, add your icing sugar and water and mix until it reaches a spreadable consistency. Carefully spread the icing over the top of your pastry layer. Immediately pipe lines of the chocolate over the icing, all in the same direction. Then, using a cocktail stick, feather the icing by lightly dragging it down in the opposite direction.

Place in the fridge to completely set. This should be overnight or no less than 6 hours. Remove from the fridge and carefully lift out of the tin, using the foil overhang.

Carefully slice through each custard slice using a sharp knife, ensuring that you cut down through the bottom layer of pastry. Some excess custard might come out around the edges which you can simply tidy up by trimming them off. Serve up immediately or keep in the fridge.

CHEESE SCONES
with Chilli Jam

 vegetarian

 low lactose — use lactose-free milk/cheese

 low fodmap — omit the chilli jam

MAKES · 8

TAKES · 30 MINUTES

- 340g / 2⅔ cups gluten-free self-raising (self-rising) flour, plus extra for dusting
- 1 tsp gluten-free baking powder
- ¼ tsp xanthan gum
- 85g / ⅓ cup plus 1 tsp cold butter, cubed
- 200g / 7oz extra mature Cheddar cheese, grated
- 2 tbsp finely chopped fresh chives
- 1½ tbsp mustard powder
- Pinch each of salt and pepper
- 180ml / ¾ cup milk
- 1 egg, beaten

Chilli Jam (makes 2 jars)

- 100g / 3½oz Bramley apple, peeled, cored and chopped
- ½ red (bell) pepper, deseeded
- 30g / 1oz red chilli peppers (medium heat), stems removed
- 500g / 2½ cups jam sugar (high pectin sugar)
- 300ml / 1¼ cups cider vinegar
- 2 tsp lemon juice

Making it dairy-free?
Use dairy-free milk and cheese and a (hard) dairy-free alternative to butter.

Making it vegan?
Follow the advice to make it dairy-free and brush with soy milk instead of egg.

As much as I love scones with jam and clotted cream, I think I might love these cheesy, savoury scones even more. Not only are they golden on the outside and fluffy in the middle, but the cheese and chive flavour combo is absolutely divine. Serve with butter and my homemade chilli jam for the ultimate experience.

Preheat your oven to 200°C fan / 220°C / 425°F. Line a large baking tray with non-stick baking parchment and place in the oven to heat up.

In a large mixing bowl, add your flour, baking powder and xanthan gum. Add your cubed butter and rub it in with your fingers until it forms a breadcrumb-like consistency. Stir in two-thirds of your cheese, the chopped chives, mustard powder, salt and pepper.

Make a well in the middle of your dry mixture, pour in the milk and mix it in using a metal spoon. Keep mixing until it all forms a dough, then use your hands to bring it together into a ball.

Lightly flour your work surface and your hands. Place your dough ball on the floured surface and fold it over a few times until smooth – don't overwork the dough. Form into a round shape about 4cm / 1½in thick (the taller the better!).

Grab a 5cm / 2in pastry cutter and use to push down into the dough, then lift the scone out with the cutter. Push the scone out of the cutter onto another area of your work surface and repeat until you've used up all of the dough. Keep re-rounding the dough and cutting to ensure you don't waste any.

Brush the tops of the scones with the beaten egg and sprinkle over the reserved cheese.

Place the scones on the heated baking tray and bake for 12–15 minutes until golden on top. Remove from the oven and transfer to a wire rack to cool slightly. Enjoy warm, or at room temperature, served with butter and my homemade chilli jam (see below), if you like.

Chilli Jam

Blitz your apple, red pepper and chilli peppers in a food processor or blender.

Place a large saucepan over a medium heat and dissolve the jam sugar in the cider vinegar and lemon juice. Once dissolved, stir in the blended pepper mixture.

Turn the heat up to medium-high and bring to an excited boil. Keep stirring constantly for 10 minutes or until the mixture is a little thicker – reduce the heat if it threatens to bubble over! Remove from the heat and allow to cool for 2–3 hours. Once cooled, serve up with your scones and store the rest in a sterilized jam jar in the fridge for up to 1 month.

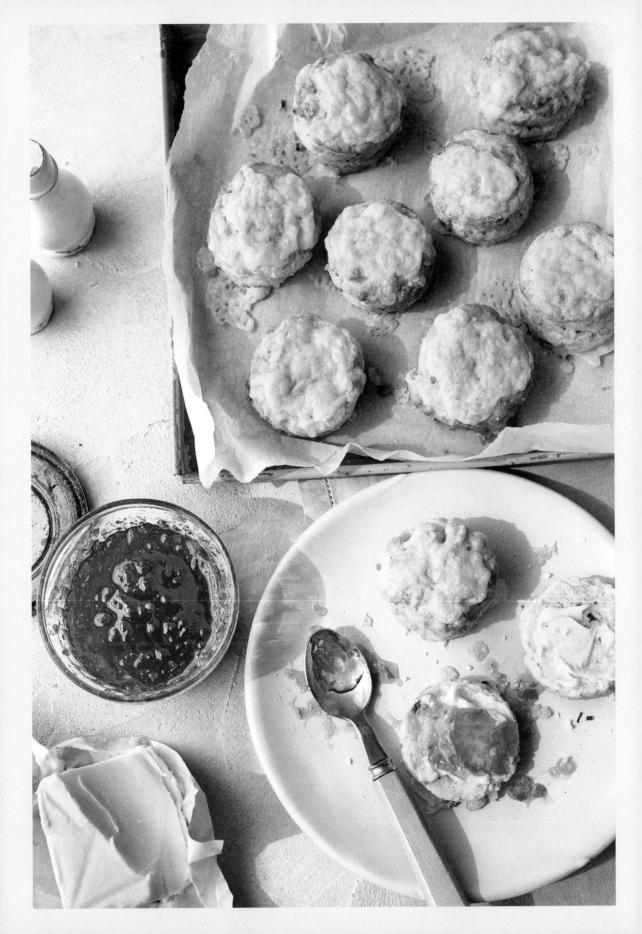

DESSERTS

I'm sure you know that feeling when it comes to ordering dessert in a restaurant. Everyone else's cheesecakes, profiteroles, pies and puddings arrive, shortly followed by your fruit salad. Of course, all gluten-free people prefer fruit for dessert... wow, sarcasm doesn't transfer well to paper, does it?

And it's that exact feeling I just described that inspired my blog and this entire chapter too. Being gluten-free shouldn't mean people assume you only like eating fruit salad, or that you should always miss out on 'the good stuff'.

So bring on my ultimate dessert menu where everything is gluten-free. I'll take a slice of one of everything, please!

NO-BAKE
Banoffee Pie

vegetarian

SERVES · 8–10

**TAKES · 45 MINUTES
+ 2 HOURS CHILLING**

For the biscuit base

- 350g / 12¼oz gluten-free digestive biscuits (graham crackers)
- 165g / ¾ cup butter, melted

For the caramel

- 1 x 397g / 14oz can (sweetened) condensed milk
- 90g / scant ½ cup light brown sugar
- 90g / ⅖ cup butter

For the topping

- 3–4 very ripe bananas
- 300ml / 1¼ cups double (heavy) cream
- 3 tbsp icing (confectioners') sugar
- A little milk chocolate, grated, to finish

This is my go-to crowd pleaser and you don't even need to turn the oven on to make it! In every bite, you're getting that buttery biscuit base, sweet, gooey caramel, tons of ripe banana, fluffy fresh cream and flakes of grated milk chocolate. Pure heaven, using just 8 ingredients.

Firstly, make your base. In a food processor, blitz your biscuits into a crumb-like texture – not into a fine dust! If you don't have a food processor, pop the biscuits into a zip-lock bag and bash them with a rolling pin.

Put your blitzed biscuits into a large bowl and pour in your melted butter. Mix until well combined. Spoon your mixture into a loose-bottomed 23cm / 9in fluted tart tin (pan). Compact the mixture into the base and up the sides of the tin using the back of a spoon. Next, press the base of a small jar or measuring cup over the biscuit base and against the sides to tightly compact, ensuring the sides are a consistent thickness. It should look deceptively similar to a pastry case.

Chill in the fridge for 30 minutes while you make your caramel.

Grab a small saucepan and place over a low heat. Add your condensed milk, sugar and butter. Allow to gently heat until melted, then stir constantly for around 10–12 minutes until thickened. Pour your caramel into the chilled biscuit base and place back in the fridge to set for 1–2 hours.

Once your caramel has set, slice your bananas into 5mm / ¼in rounds and place over the caramel in one or two layers.

In a mixing bowl, either by hand or using a stand mixer or electric hand whisk, whip your cream and icing sugar until it forms soft peaks. Spoon the cream over the bananas and finish with a little grated chocolate. Return the pie to the fridge until ready to serve.

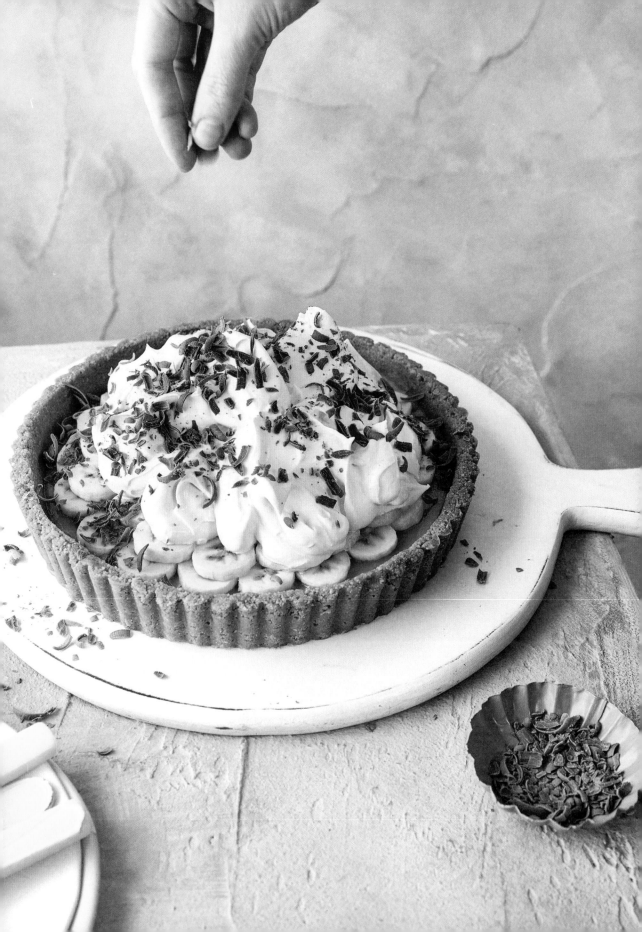

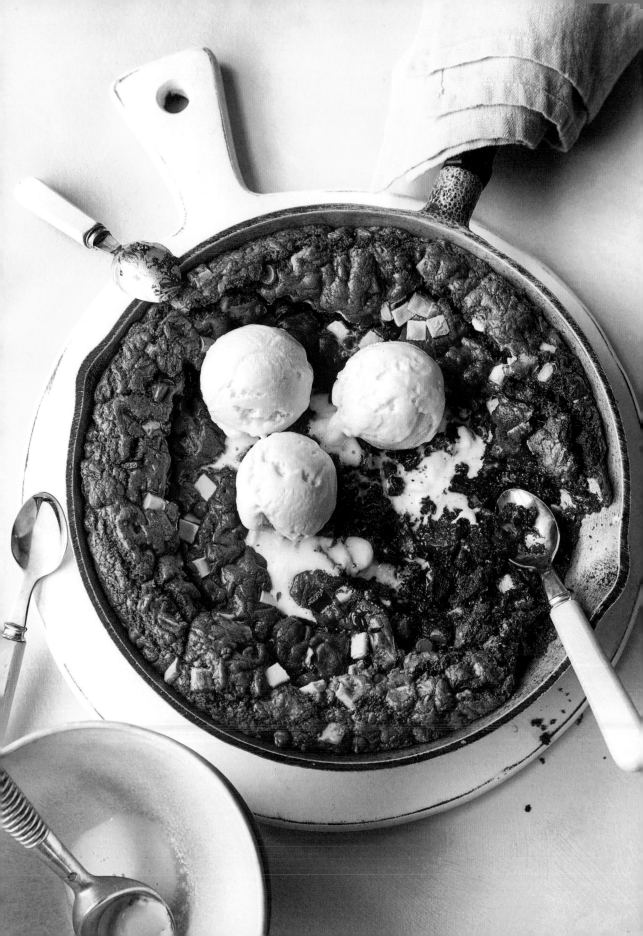

Triple Chocolate
COOKIE DOUGH SKILLET

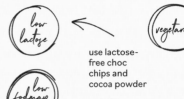

low lactose

vegetarian

low fodmap

use lactose-free choc chips and cocoa powder

SERVES · 5–6

TAKES · 45 MINUTES

- 120g / generous ½ cup butter, melted, plus extra for greasing
- 100g / ½ cup caster (superfine) sugar
- 100g / ½ cup light brown sugar
- 1 large egg
- 1 tsp vanilla extract
- 200g / 1½ cups gluten-free plain (all-purpose) flour
- 1 tsp bicarbonate of soda (baking soda)
- 25g / ¼ cup cocoa powder
- 250g / 9oz mixed chocolate chips (white, dark and milk)

Graduate to true gluten-free 'cookie monster' status with my crisp on the outside, gooey in the middle, triple chocolate cookie dough skillet. Serve with vanilla ice cream and thank me later.

Preheat your oven to 160°C fan / 180°C / 350°F. Grease a skillet or 20cm / 8in round cake tin (pan) with a little butter.

You can happily use an electric hand mixer to make your cookie dough, but I prefer to do this one by hand. In a large mixing bowl, add your melted butter and both sugars. Mix until really well combined and slightly stiff.

Add your egg and vanilla and mix until fully combined. Next, sift in your flour, bicarb and cocoa powder. Mix in thoroughly until you have a smooth, thick cookie dough. Mix in your chocolate chips, then evenly spoon your mixture into your skillet or tin. You can push a few extra chocolate chips in the top if there aren't many showing already.

Bake in the oven for 30 minutes until the top is cooked but still gooey underneath. Allow to cool for 15 minutes. If you like it a bit less gooey in the middle, leave it a little longer to cool. Enjoy straight from the skillet with vanilla ice cream.

TIP:
You can also reheat a portion by giving it a quick blast in the microwave.

Making it dairy-free?
Use a (hard) dairy-free alternative to butter and dairy-free chocolate chips. Ensure the cocoa powder is dairy-free too.

Making it vegan?
Follow the advice to make it dairy-free, then replace the egg with 3 tbsp aquafaba (whisked until frothy).

Churros

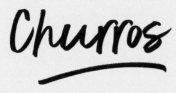

 use dairy-free milk and chocolate and a hard dairy-free butter alternative

 use lactose-free milk and chocolate

 use lactose-free milk and chocolate

SERVES · 4

TAKES · 45 MINUTES

- 250ml / 1 cup water
- 60g / ¼ cup butter
- 20g / 1½ tbsp caster (superfine) sugar
- 135g / 1 cup gluten-free plain (all-purpose) flour
- ¼ tsp xanthan gum
- ½ tsp vanilla extract
- 1 egg, beaten
- Vegetable oil, for frying

For the sugar coating

- 100g / ½ cup caster (superfine) sugar
- 1 tsp ground cinnamon

For the chocolate dipping sauce

- 100g / 3½oz dark chocolate
- 75ml / 5 tbsp milk
- 2 tbsp maple syrup

I never had the pleasure of enjoying churros when I could still eat gluten, but I'm more than making up for it now! They're basically like little fried doughnut sticks - super crisp on the outside and fluffy in the middle. Dip in my 3-ingredient chocolate sauce and enjoy!

Add your water, butter and sugar to a large saucepan and place over a low heat. Allow to melt, stirring until well combined, then bring to a very gentle boil and remove from the heat. Add your flour and xanthan gum and immediately stir well to remove any potential lumps. Keep stirring until well combined.

Grab a large mixing bowl, add your warm dough and allow the mixture to cool for 10 minutes, then stir in your vanilla and gradually add in your beaten egg, stirring between each addition (I use an electric hand whisk for this part). Whisk until smooth and consistent. You might not need all the egg, so stop when it reaches a lovely, thick, pipeable consistency.

Grab a large, heavy-based saucepan, place over a medium heat and add vegetable oil to a depth of 4cm / 1½in. Heat for around 10 minutes until the oil reaches 170°C / 340°F - test with a cooking thermometer or use the wooden spoon handle test (page 19).

While the oil is heating, make your chocolate dipping sauce. Grab a small saucepan and place over a low heat. Add your chocolate, milk and maple syrup and allow to melt down. Stir until well until combined and keep warm.

Prepare a piping bag using a medium-sized, open star nozzle. Spoon as much of your dough into the piping bag as will comfortably fit.

Once your oil has reached the desired temperature, working in batches, pipe your dough directly into the oil in smooth 15cm / 6in lines, snipping off each piped churro using a pair of kitchen scissors to separate them. Cook for 2 minutes, then turn over and cook for a further 2 minutes, until nice and golden on both sides, then remove from the oil using a slotted spoon and place on some kitchen paper to drain.

Mix your sugar and cinnamon in a shallow dish until well combined and coat your warm churros in the mixture. Serve with the chocolate sauce for dipping.

TIP:
Churros are freezer-friendly! Simply pipe any excess dough onto a baking tray lined with non-stick baking parchment and place in the freezer. Then, whenever you fancy churros, simply pop them into the hot oil straight from frozen and cook them for 30 seconds more on each side.

Making it vegan?
Use dairy-free milk, dairy-free chocolate and a (hard) dairy-free alternative to butter. Replace the egg with 3 tbsp aquafaba (whisked until frothy).

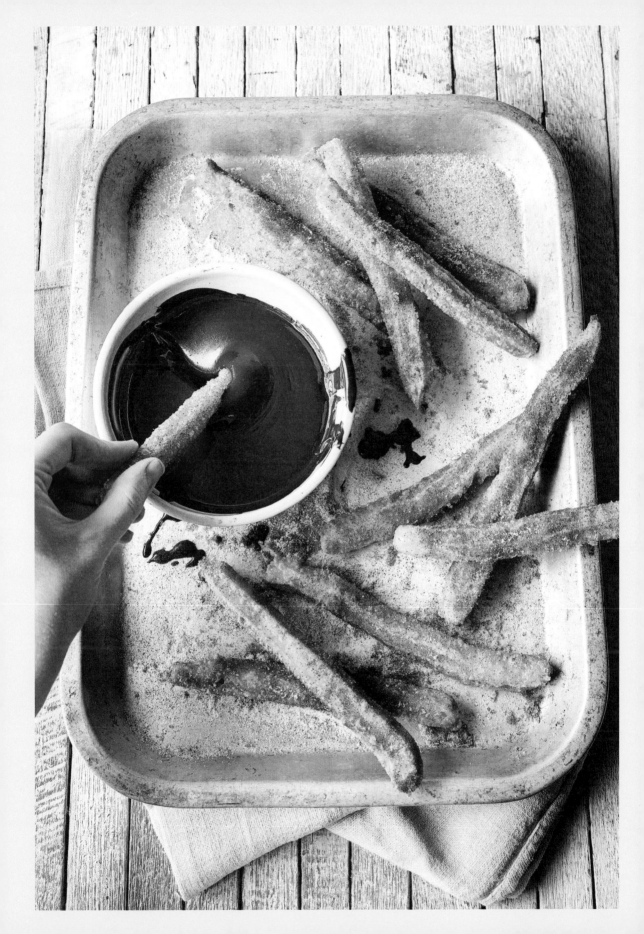

Salted Caramel
NO-BAKE CHEESECAKE

vegetarian

SERVES · 10–12

**TAKES · 45 MINUTES
+ 12 HOURS CHILLING**

For the biscuit base

- 320g / 11¼oz gluten-free digestive biscuits (graham crackers)
- 2 tbsp light brown sugar
- 150g / ⅔ cup butter, melted

For the cheesecake filling

- 700g / generous 3 cups full-fat cream cheese or mascarpone
- 100g / scant ¾ cup icing (confectioners') sugar
- Pinch of salt
- 3–4 tsp caramel extract
- 300ml / 1¼ cups double (heavy) cream
- 150g / 5¼oz gluten-free chocolate-covered caramels (optional)

To serve

- 200g / 7oz caramel sauce (ensure gluten-free), with a pinch of salt added
- Toffee popcorn (optional)

It couldn't be easier to whip up this no-bake show-stopper – no oven or gluten-free flour required! With a buttery biscuit base, indulgent caramel filling, topped with caramel sauce, this is the dessert that we all deserve after years of fruit salad.

Firstly, make your base. In a food processor, blitz your biscuits into a crumb-like texture – not into a fine dust! If you don't have a food processor, pop the biscuits into a zip-lock bag and bash them with a rolling pin. Add to a large mixing bowl with the sugar and pour in your melted butter. Mix until well combined.

Spoon into a round 20cm / 8in loose-bottomed or springform tin (pan). Compact the mixture into the base to create a nice, even layer. Chill in the fridge for 30 minutes while you make your filling.

For the filling, place your cream cheese, icing sugar, salt and caramel extract in a stand mixer. Mix on a low–medium speed for 10–20 seconds. Add the cream and, at a medium speed, mix for 2 more minutes or until the mixture begins to firm up. Don't over-mix it as the mixture can split and then won't set in the fridge. It should end up as a nice, thick, spoonable mixture, not a pourable consistency. At this point, you can also fold in some chopped up chocolate-covered caramels by hand, if using.

(You can of course make the cheesecake filling using an electric hand whisk too. Also, while making the cheesecake filling by hand requires a little extra time and elbow grease, it's more than possible! I'd recommend sifting your icing sugar first if making it by hand.)

Next, evenly spread your cheesecake filling on top of the chilled biscuit base and place in the fridge to chill for a minimum of 12 hours, ideally overnight.

When you're ready to serve, remove the cheesecake from the tin and decorate by carefully pouring your salted caramel sauce on top to form a thin layer. Finish decorating with some toffee popcorn, if you like.

TIP:
This is freezer-friendly! Once the cheesecake has set, place it in the freezer whole or sliced. Defrost thoroughly before topping with the caramel sauce and toffee popcorn.

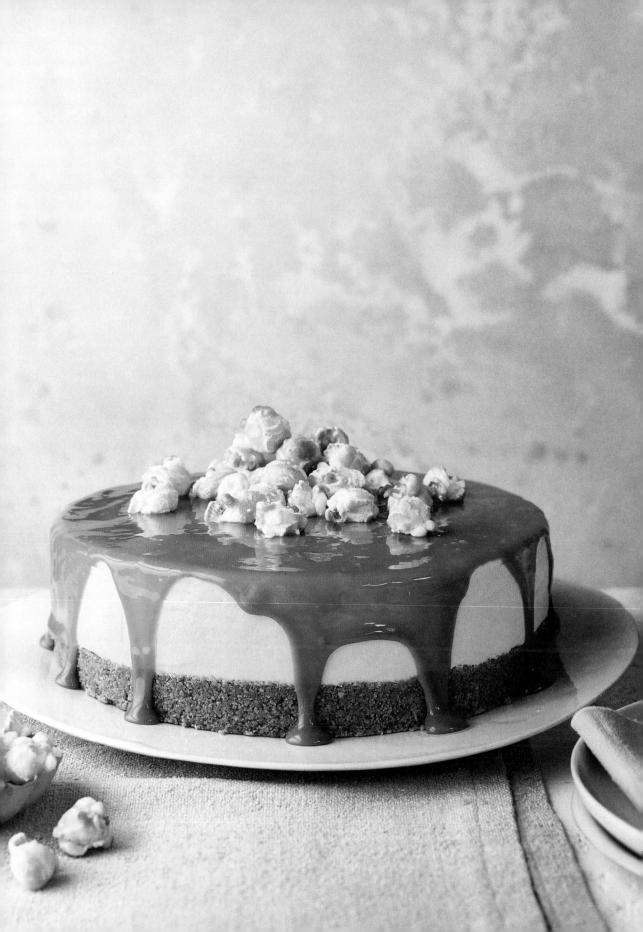

· NEW YORK ·
Baked Cheesecake

vegetarian

SERVES · 10–12

**TAKES · 1 HOUR
+ 12 HOURS CHILLING**

For the base
- 320g / 11¼oz gluten-free digestive biscuits (graham crackers)
- 150g / ⅔ cup butter, melted

For the cheesecake filling
- 600g / 2⅔ cups full-fat cream cheese
- 30g / 2½ tbsp gluten-free plain (all-purpose) flour
- 185g / scant 2 cups caster (superfine) sugar
- 3 eggs, beaten
- 2 tsp vanilla extract
- Grated zest of ½ lemon plus 2 tsp juice (optional)
- 175g / ¾ cup sour cream

Sometimes, only a perfectly baked cheesecake will do! The buttery biscuit base somehow tastes even better after baking, and the filling... just wow. It has an incredibly creamy texture with a sweet vanilla flavour that you just can't get in a no-bake cheesecake.

Firstly, make your base. In a food processor, blitz your biscuits into a crumb-like texture – not into a fine dust! If you don't have a food processor, pop the biscuits into a zip-lock bag and bash them with a rolling pin. Add to a large mixing bowl and pour in your melted butter. Mix until well combined.

Spoon into a round 20cm / 8in loose-bottomed or springform tin (pan). Compact the mixture into the base to create a nice, even layer. Chill in the fridge for 30 minutes while you make your cheesecake filling.

Preheat your oven to 200°C fan / 220°C / 425°F.

For the filling, place your cream cheese in a stand mixer and mix on a low speed for 1 minute. In a small bowl, mix your flour and sugar together, then gradually add this to your mixer, maintaining the low speed. Next, gradually add your beaten eggs along with the vanilla and lemon zest and juice, if using. Fold in your sour cream by hand.

(You can of course make the cheesecake filling using an electric hand whisk too. Also, while making the cheesecake filling by hand requires a little extra time and elbow grease, it's more than possible!)

Next, evenly spread your filling on top of the chilled biscuit base, bake in the oven for 10 minutes, then reduce the oven temperature to 90°C fan / 110°C / 225°F and bake for a further 30–35 minutes. When cooked, it should be wobbly and a little brown around the edges, but instead of removing it from the oven, leave it in, turn the oven off and keep the door shut for another 30 minutes.

After 30 minutes, leave the door of the oven ajar to allow the cheesecake to cool slowly (this will prevent cracking in the top). Leave to cool for 2–3 hours. Once cooled, cover in foil (around the edges and underneath the tin too), then place in the fridge to chill for 12 hours, ideally overnight.

When you're ready to serve, remove the cheesecake from the tin and slice.

TIP:
This is freezer-friendly! You can freeze this as a whole cheesecake or in individual slices.

Jam
ROLY-POLY

use a hard dairy-free butter alternative and dairy-free milk

use lactose-free milk

SERVES · 5

TAKES · 1 HOUR

- A little softened butter, for greasing
- 180g / 1⅓ cups gluten-free self-raising (self-rising) flour, plus extra for dusting
- ¼ tsp xanthan gum
- 20g / 1½ tbsp cold butter, cubed
- 25g / 2 tbsp caster (superfine) sugar
- 80g / ⅔ cup gluten-free vegetable suet
- 115ml / scant ½ cup milk
- Raspberry jam (jelly)

This classic British pudding is soft, delightfully stodgy, packed with sticky jam and perfect with lashings of custard. Finding a gluten-free version is next to impossible, so I'm sure you know what to do next!

Preheat your oven to 180°C fan / 200°C / 400°F. Place a roasting dish in the bottom of the oven and boil a kettle.

Cut a sheet of non-stick baking parchment and a sheet of foil to 35 x 30cm / 14 x 12in. Layer the baking parchment on top of the foil and grease the top of the baking parchment using softened butter. Set aside.

In a large bowl, mix your flour and xanthan gum. Add your diced butter and rub it in with your fingers until it forms a breadcrumb-like consistency, then stir in your sugar and suet.

Gradually mix in your milk – I use a knife to cut this into the mixture. At this point, it should start to come together and begin to form a dough. Bring it together with your hands into a ball. Dough too sticky? Just add a small amount of extra flour to the dough.

On a sheet of lightly floured baking parchment, roll out your dough into a rectangle, roughly 32 x 22cm / 12½ x 8½in. Spread a layer of jam all over the dough, leaving a 2cm / ¾in border along one of the short edges.

Very carefully and tightly roll the dough up from the opposite shorter edge, towards the end where you left the clear border. Seal the rolled up roly-poly by pinching the dough together along the seam to prevent the jam leaking out. Place on the greased parchment with the foil beneath. Bring the parchment and foil up and over the roly-poly and loosely seal like a wrapped parcel. Give it lots of room as it will expand in the oven.

Next, add a mug's worth of boiling water to your preheated roasting dish (pull the dish out of the oven a little and pour in, no need to remove it). Place your jam roly-poly on the rack above the roasting dish and cook for 45 minutes.

Once cooked, allow the roly-poly to sit in the foil and parchment for about 5 minutes before opening. Slice and serve hot with my quick, thick gluten-free custard (page 37) and some extra jam.

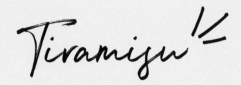

Tiramisu

SERVES · 4–6

**TAKES · 15 MINUTES
+ 3–4 HOURS CHILLING**

- 300ml / 1¼ cups freshly made strong black coffee
- 2 tbsp coffee liqueur, brandy or Marsala (optional)
- 250ml / 1 cup double (heavy) cream
- 70g / 6 tbsp caster (superfine) sugar
- 1 tsp vanilla extract
- 250g / 1 cup full-fat mascarpone cheese
- 12 gluten-free ladyfingers (page 31 or use store-bought gluten-free sponge cakes)
- 50g / 1¾oz dark chocolate, grated, plus extra to serve
- 3 tbsp cocoa powder

When we last went to Rome, I was surrounded by gluten-free tiramisu. Back at home, I'd sooner spot a unicorn. So I decided to make my own! (gluten-free tiramisu, not a unicorn). It's bursting with that deep, rich coffee flavour, with the bitterness offset by sweet, creamy mascarpone.

Pour your coffee into a small bowl and add in your liqueur, if using. Set aside to cool.

Whip together your cream, sugar and vanilla until soft peaks form. Add in your mascarpone and mix together until combined and the mixture is slightly stiffer. (I use an electric hand whisk for this.)

Once your coffee has cooled, one at a time, dip your ladyfingers into it for no more than a second on each side, or they will get very soggy.

Place a layer of soaked fingers in the base of a dish, about 33 x 23cm / 13 x 9in. Try to fill all the gaps by breaking some up into smaller pieces if necessary. Spread half of your cream mixture over the ladyfingers, then sprinkle the grated chocolate evenly on top of the cream. Repeat with another layer of ladyfingers, then the rest of the cream. Sift over the cocoa powder and place in the fridge to chill for at least 3–4 hours.

Serve straight from the fridge with a little extra grated chocolate on top to finish it off.

TIP:
If you want to make this into a bigger dish to serve more people, then simply double the ingredients accordingly.

Caramel
PROFITEROLES

MAKES · 18

**TAKES · 45 MINUTES
+ 2 HOURS COOLING**

- 1 quantity of gluten-free choux pastry (page 30)
- 40ml / 3 tbsp caramel sauce (ensure gluten-free), to serve

For the crème pâtissière filling

- 450ml / generous 1¾ cups whole milk
- 1½ tsp caramel extract (vanilla extract would be fine too)
- 150g / ¾ cup caster (superfine) sugar
- 40g / 2 tbsp cornflour (cornstarch)
- 2 whole eggs plus 2 egg yolks

For the chocolate ganache

- 175ml / ¾ cup double (heavy) cream
- 175g / 6¼oz dark or milk chocolate, finely chopped

This recipe is absolutely inspired by my dad, who (several million times a year) would go into great detail about the miraculous caramel profiteroles he once enjoyed while away on a business trip. So of course, I grilled him about them, then made them so that we could both enjoy them together. They're packed with a lovely caramel cream and topped with chocolate ganache and a caramel sauce. Now I know what all the fuss was about!

Start by making the crème pâtissière filling. In a large saucepan, heat the milk and caramel extract together over a medium heat until just before it begins to boil.

In a large mixing bowl, add the sugar, cornflour, eggs and egg yolks and whisk until well combined and slightly paler.

Gradually pour the hot milk into your mixing bowl, whisking in between each addition. Keep whisking continuously until it's all combined. Pour the mixture back into your saucepan and place over a medium heat. Whisk for around 5 minutes until the mixture thickens. Once thickened, continue whisking for 2 minutes, then remove from the heat. Transfer to a clean bowl. If you notice any lumps in your custard – don't worry! You can always sieve it into the bowl.

Cover with cling film (plastic wrap) so that it is touching the surface of the custard; this will prevent a skin from forming as it cools. Place in the fridge for 2–3 hours to completely cool and further thicken.

Preheat your oven to 200°C fan / 220°C / 425°F. Line a large baking sheet with non-stick baking parchment.

Transfer your choux pastry dough to a piping bag fitted with an open star nozzle. If you don't have a piping bag, you can simply spoon it onto the baking tray instead.

Pipe balls that are 5cm / 2in in diameter onto your baking tray, leaving a 2cm / ¾in space between each ball to allow for them to puff out in the oven. Wet your finger and dab the top of each ball to help round them off, gently smoothing over any pointy bits.

Bake in the oven for 25 minutes, reducing the oven temperature after 15 minutes to 150°C fan / 170°C / 340°F, until puffy and golden. Never open the oven until they are ready to be taken out!

Remove from the oven and, using a skewer, pierce the bottom of each one and place upside down in order to let the steam out – this will prevent them from becoming soggy inside. Allow to slowly cool down on the baking tray in the oven, turned off with the door ajar, for 20 minutes. Then transfer to a wire rack to fully cool.

Once your profiteroles are cool and your filling is prepared, you have two choices of how to fill them. Firstly, you can carefully slice the profiteroles in half and spoon (or pipe) the filling in as though you were assembling a sandwich. Alternatively, you can place your crème pâtissière in a piping bag with a long filler nozzle and pipe it in from the bottom of the profiterole until it starts to feel heavier and full.

For your chocolate ganache top, pour your cream into a saucepan and heat until just before it begins to boil. Add your chopped chocolate to a heatproof bowl and pour the hot cream onto the chocolate. Leave to stand for a few minutes before mixing together until smooth. Briefly cool and then dip the top of your profiteroles into the ganache.

Drizzle with your caramel sauce just before serving. Enjoy immediately before the pastry starts to lose its crisp exterior, or store in the fridge for 1–2 hours.

TIPS:
If you wish to keep them longer, store unfilled in an airtight container for up to 2 days. Then simply warm them in the oven at 200°C fan / 220°C / 425°F for 5 minutes, allow to cool and proceed with the rest of the recipe.

If you're in a hurry, you can always use the fresh cream filling used in my chocolate éclairs on page 204.

Pictured on page 205

Making it dairy-free?
Use dairy-free milk for the crème pâtissière. Top with melted dairy-free chocolate instead of chocolate ganache and use a dairy-free caramel – there's a recipe on my blog if you need one!

Making it lactose-free?
Or low FODMAP?
Use lactose-free milk for the crème pâtissière. Top with melted lactose-free chocolate instead of chocolate ganache. Omit the caramel sauce.

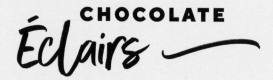

CHOCOLATE
Éclairs

vegetarian

MAKES · 14

TAKES · 45 MINUTES

- 1 quantity of gluten-free choux pastry (page 30)
- 200ml / generous ¾ cup double (heavy) cream
- 4 tsp icing (confectioners') sugar
- 1 tsp vanilla extract

For the chocolate ganache

- 175ml / ¾ cup double (heavy) cream
- 175g / 6¼oz dark or milk chocolate, finely chopped

Fortunately for us, gluten-free choux pastry is incredibly easy to make and absolutely indistinguishable from its gluten equivalent. So, naturally, my éclairs are lovely and crisp on the outside, packed with tons of fresh cream and topped with chocolate ganache. Exactly how they should be!

Preheat your oven to 200°C fan / 220°C / 425°F. Line a large baking sheet with non-stick baking parchment.

Transfer your choux pastry dough to a piping bag fitted with an open star nozzle. If you don't have a piping bag, you can simply spoon it onto the baking tray instead. Pipe thick, straight lines, 10cm / 4in long, onto your baking sheet, leaving space between them as they will puff up when baked.

Bake in the oven for 25 minutes, reducing the oven temperature after 15 minutes to 150°C fan / 170°C / 340°F, until puffy and golden. Never open the oven until they are ready to be taken out!

Remove from the oven and, using a skewer, pierce the bottom of each one three times and place upside down in order to let the steam out – this will prevent them from becoming soggy inside. Allow to slowly cool down on the baking tray in the oven, turned off with the door ajar, for 20 minutes. Then transfer to a wire rack to fully cool.

For the filling, grab a large mixing bowl. Add your cream, icing sugar and vanilla and whisk until it forms fairly stiff peaks. Be careful not to over-whisk it.

Once your éclairs are cool and your filling is prepared, you have two choices of how to fill them. Firstly, you can carefully slice the éclairs in half and spoon (or pipe) the filling on as though you were assembling a sandwich. Alternatively, you can place your cream filling in a piping bag fitted with a long filler nozzle and pipe the cream in from the bottom of the éclair until it starts to feel heavier and full.

For your chocolate ganache top, pour your cream into a saucepan and heat until just before it begins to boil. Add the chopped chocolate to a heatproof bowl and pour the hot cream into the bowl. Leave to stand for a few minutes before mixing together until smooth.

Briefly cool, then dip the top of your éclairs into the ganache.

Enjoy immediately before the pastry starts to lose its crisp exterior, or store in the fridge for 1–2 hours.

TIPS:
If you wish to keep your éclairs for longer, store unfilled in an airtight container for up to 2 days. Then, simply warm them in the oven at 200°C fan / 220°C / 425°F for 5 minutes, allow to cool and proceed with the rest of the recipe.

If you'd prefer, fill your éclairs with the caramel crème pâtissière on page 202.

Making it dairy-free?
Instead of filling with fresh cream, use the crème pâtissière on page 202 and make it with dairy-free milk. Top with melted dairy-free chocolate instead of chocolate ganache.

Making it lactose-free?
Or low FODMAP?
Instead of filling with fresh cream, use the crème pâtissière on page 202 and make it with lactose-free milk. Top with melted lactose-free chocolate instead of chocolate ganache.

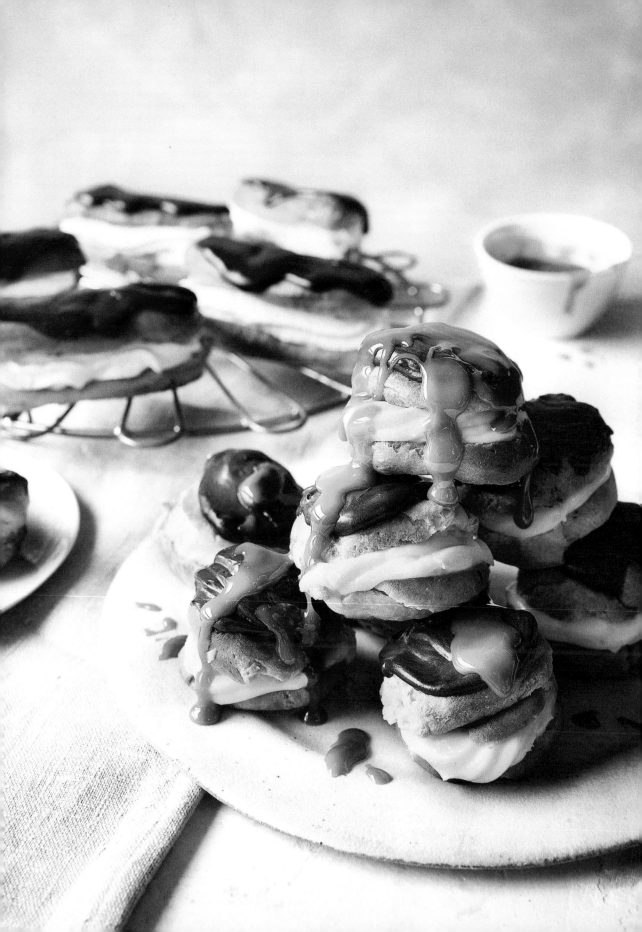

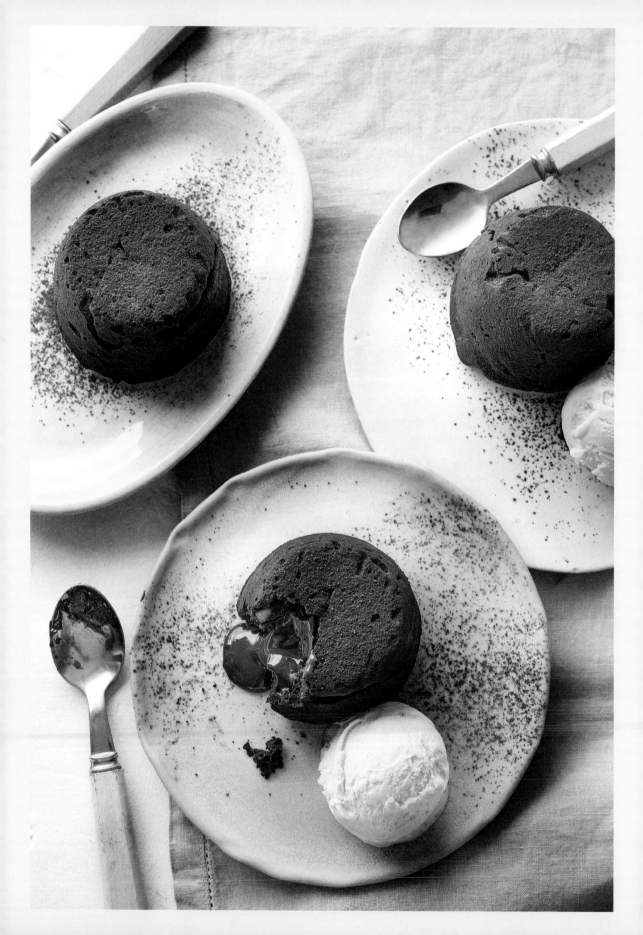

Chocolate
FONDANTS

 use a hard dairy-free butter alternative, dairy-free chocolate and cocoa powder

 ensure chocolate and cocoa powder are lactose-free

 ensure chocolate and cocoa powder are lactose-free

SERVES · 5

TAKES · 30 MINUTES

For the mini pudding moulds
- 10g / ¾ tbsp butter, melted
- Cocoa powder, for dusting

For the chocolate fondant
- 200g / 7oz dark chocolate, broken into pieces
- 100g / ½ cup minus 1 tbsp butter
- 100g / ½ cup caster (superfine) sugar
- 3 eggs, plus 2 egg yolks
- 50g / 6 tbsp gluten-free plain (all-purpose) flour
- 50g / 1¾oz finely chopped hazelnuts (optional)

These soft little fondants are packed with a gooey, melting middle and are so easy to make. I love adding chopped hazelnuts too, which give them a lovely chocolate-hazelnut flavour! You'll need 5 mini pudding moulds to make these, FYI.

Begin by preparing your mini pudding moulds. Brush the melted butter over the insides of the moulds then sift a little cocoa powder into each one and rotate to coat the sides and base. Place in the freezer to chill while you make the fondant mixture.

Melt together your chocolate and butter. You can do this two ways: in the microwave, making sure you stir every 20–30 seconds until fully melted, or in a heatproof bowl placed over a saucepan of gently boiling water, making sure the water isn't touching the base of the bowl. Keep stirring until everything has melted and mixed together. Put to one side and allow to cool briefly.

In a large mixing bowl, whisk your sugar, eggs and egg yolks until slightly thickened and frothy (I use an electric hand whisk for this). Gradually add your slightly cooled chocolate and butter mixture to the bowl. Fold in gently, then fold in your flour, and chopped hazelnuts if using, until well combined.

Remove your pudding moulds from the freezer. Pour your fondant mixture into a jug (pitcher) then evenly divide between your moulds, leaving a 1cm / ⅜in gap at the top of each. Place in the fridge to chill for 30 minutes (or up to 6 hours). Preheat your oven to 180°C fan / 200°C / 400°F.

Place your chilled moulds on a baking sheet and bake in the oven for 13–15 minutes, until risen up with a nicely set top. Remove from the oven and leave the fondants to sit in their moulds for about 1 minute before inverting them onto plates to serve. Enjoy with vanilla ice cream.

TIP:
These are freezer-friendly! Freeze the mixture in the moulds, ready to bake from frozen. Simply add 5 minutes to the cooking time.

Creamy Lemon
TART

vegetarian

SERVES · 8

**TAKES · 1 HOUR
+ 1 HOUR CHILLING**

- 1 quantity of gluten-free shortcrust pastry (page 27), chilled for 25 minutes
- Gluten-free plain (all-purpose) flour, for dusting
- Fresh raspberries, to serve

For the filling

- 700g / 1lb 8½oz (sweetened) condensed milk
- 4 egg yolks
- Grated zest and juice of 4 large lemons (160ml / ⅔ cup juice)

Gone are the days where I can buy a lemon tart with a sweet, creamy, zesty filling, encased in light, buttery pastry. But actually, making your own at home is not only incredibly simple, it tastes a million miles better than what I used to buy anyway! Once you've made your pastry, you only need three simple ingredients to make the filling.

Remove your pastry from the fridge. If it feels really firm when you take it out, leave it out at room temperature briefly before rolling it. Don't handle your dough excessively as this will warm it up and make it more fragile.

Lightly flour your rolling pin. On a sheet of non-stick baking parchment, roll out the dough to a large circle 3mm /⅛in thick. Transfer the pastry to a 23cm / 9in fluted tart tin (pan) by supporting the pastry as you gently invert it into the tin, with equal overhang on all sides. Peel off the parchment.

Next, use your fingers to carefully ease the pastry into place, so that it neatly lines the tin. Lift the overhanging pastry and, using your thumb, squash 2mm / ¹⁄₁₆in of pastry back into the tin. This will result in slightly thicker sides, which will prevent your pastry case from shrinking when baked. Allow the overhang to do its thing – we'll trim it after chilling it.

Lightly prick the base of the pastry case with a fork, then place in the fridge for 15 minutes. Preheat the oven to 180°C fan / 200°C / 400°F and place a large baking tray in the oven to heat up.

After chilling, use a rolling pin to roll over the top of the tart tin, removing the overhang and flattening down the pastry. Loosely line the base of the pastry case with baking parchment and fill with baking beans (or uncooked rice if you don't have any). Bake on the heated baking tray in the oven for 15 minutes, then remove the baking parchment and baking beans and bake for a further 5 minutes. Remove from the oven and allow to fully cool. Reduce the oven temperature to 160°C fan / 180°C / 350°F.

In a large mixing bowl, mix all the filling ingredients together until smooth (I use an electric hand whisk for this). Pour the mixture into your cooled pastry case, ensuring it's nice and level. Bake in the oven for 20 minutes until the filling is firm with a very slight wobble. Allow to cool to room temperature before placing it in the fridge to firm up for at least an hour.

Serve with fresh raspberries, or if you're feeling adventurous, use your leftover egg whites to make some Italian meringue for the top.

TIP:
If you don't have time to make your own pastry, use store-bought gluten-free pastry instead.

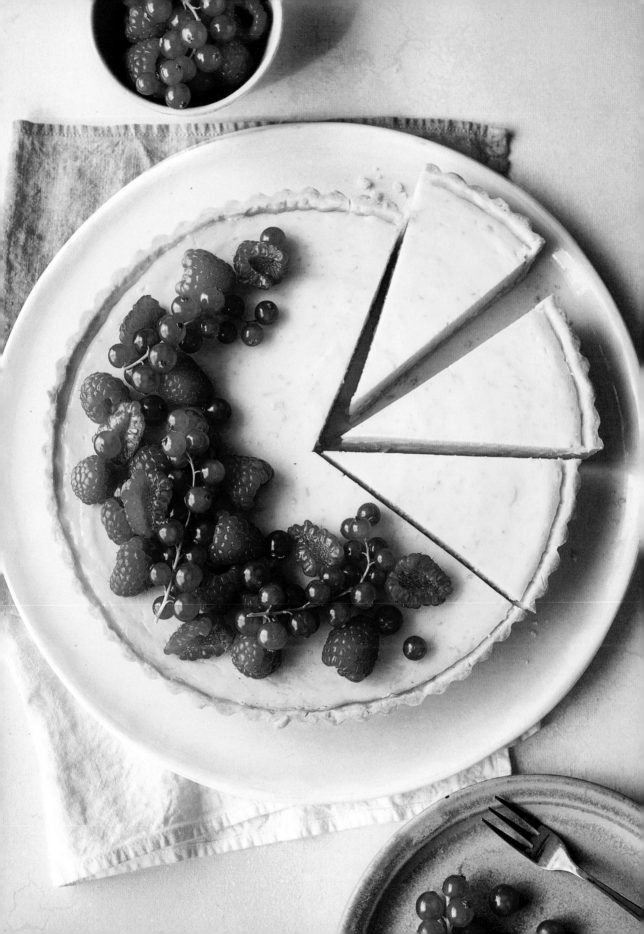

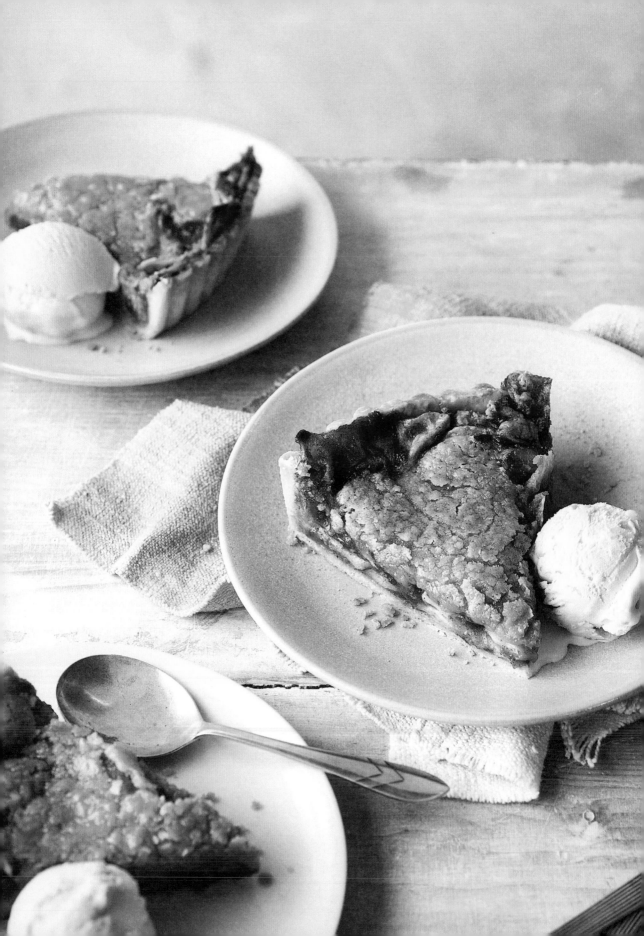

APPLE CRUMBLE *Pie*

use a hard dairy-free butter alternative

SERVES · 8–10

TAKES · 1 HOUR

- 1 quantity of gluten-free shortcrust pastry (page 27), chilled for 25 minutes
- Gluten-free plain (all-purpose) flour, for dusting

For the filling

- 80g / 6½ tbsp light brown sugar
- 15g / 1 tbsp butter
- 600g / 1lb 5oz Bramley apples, peeled, cored and sliced into short 5mm / ¼in slices
- 1 tsp ground cinnamon
- 2 tsp lemon juice
- 2 tbsp cornflour (cornstarch)

For the crumble topping

- 85g / 7 tbsp light brown sugar
- 100g / ¾ cup gluten-free plain (all-purpose) flour
- 1 tsp vanilla extract
- 85g / generous ⅓ cup butter, melted and cooled

I decided to combine my two favourite desserts for this one: an apple pie and an apple crumble. And I'm so glad I did! With buttery pastry, tons of sticky, thinly sliced apple, topped with a crispy, crunchy, crumble topping, this pie is almost too good to share.

Remove your chilled pastry from the fridge. If it feels really firm when you take it out, leave it out at room temperature briefly before rolling it. Don't handle your dough excessively as this will warm it up and make it more fragile.

Lightly flour your rolling pin. On a sheet of non-stick baking parchment, roll out the pastry into a large circle, 3mm / ⅛in thick. Transfer to a 23cm / 9in fluted tart tin (pan), by supporting the pastry as you gently invert it into the tin, with equal overhang on all sides. Peel off the baking parchment.

Next, use your fingers to carefully ease the pastry into place so that it neatly lines the tin. Lift the overhanging pastry and, using your thumb, squash 2mm / ¹⁄₁₆in of pastry back into the tin. This will result in slightly thicker sides, which will prevent your pastry case from shrinking when baked. Allow the overhang to do its thing – we'll trim the overhang after chilling it.

Lightly prick the base of the pastry case with a fork, then place it in the fridge for 15 minutes. Preheat the oven to 180°C fan / 200°C / 400°F and place a baking tray inside to heat up.

After chilling, use a rolling pin to roll over the top of the tin, removing the overhang and flattening down the pastry. Loosely line the base of the pastry case with baking parchment and fill with baking beans (or uncooked rice if you don't have any). Bake in the oven on the heated tray

for 15 minutes, then remove the parchment and beans and bake for a further 5 minutes. Remove from the oven and allow to fully cool.

Next, prepare your crumble topping. In a bowl, mix your sugar, flour, vanilla and cooled melted butter together until well combined, then chill in the fridge until needed.

Now prepare your pie filling. Place a large saucepan over a low heat and add your brown sugar and butter. Allow to fully melt before adding your apples, cinnamon and lemon juice. Mix to coat the apples and gently simmer until some of the juices begin to appear. Sift in your cornflour and immediately mix to ensure it doesn't go lumpy. Continue to cook your apples until the juices thicken and the apples are ever so slightly softened. You don't want them to be mushy! Remove from the heat and allow to cool slightly.

To construct the pie, spoon your apple filling into the pastry case. There shouldn't be any thin juices, just the thickened juices as a result of the cornflour. Sprinkle chunks of the chilled crumble all over the top of the apples. Bake in the oven for 30 minutes or until the crumble top is golden.

Serve with vanilla ice cream or my quick thick custard (page 37).

TIP:
If you don't have time to make your own pastry, use store-bought gluten-free pastry instead.

Auntie Carol's
TRIFLE

SERVES · 5–6

TAKES · 10 MINUTES

- 6–8 gluten-free ladyfingers (page 31 or use store-bought gluten-free sponge cakes)
- 50g / 1¾oz raspberry or strawberry jam (jelly)
- 50–100ml / 3½–7 tbsp dry sherry (or orange juice to make it alcohol-free)
- 200g / 7oz frozen strawberries and raspberries
- 1 large banana, sliced
- 500ml / 2 cups thick gluten-free custard (page 37 or store-bought)
- 300ml / 1¼ cups double (heavy) cream
- 2 tbsp icing (confectioners') sugar
- Flaked (slivered) almonds or grated chocolate, to sprinkle

My Auntie Carol and Uncle Neil always used to turn up for family dinners with this absolutely enormous, beautiful trifle. It's been a long time since I've been able to eat it, but fortunately, my aunt gave me her recipe so I could adapt it and share it with all of you. It's every bit as good as I remember, with tons of jammy sponge, thick custard and heaps of whipped cream. I used a 2-litre trifle bowl to make this, FYI.

Break your ladyfingers into slightly smaller pieces and spread a little jam on half of them. Sandwich them together with the other halves and arrange in your trifle dish to cover the entire base.

Next, pour over your sherry (or orange juice) and allow it to soak into the ladyfingers. Sprinkle your frozen berries over the top and push them in a little, then add your sliced banana. Pour the custard over the top.

Whip the cream with the icing sugar until thickened, and spoon on top of your custard.

Finish with some flaked almonds or grated chocolate.

Allow to set and chill in the fridge until ready to serve.

TIP:
You could also use my Swiss roll (page 171) instead of ladyfingers for the base. Simply make the Swiss roll with a jammy filling – it can look absolutely awesome when pressed up against the sides of your trifle dish.

Making it dairy-free?
Make my quick, thick custard (page 37) using dairy-free milk and a coconut whipping cream instead of double cream. Use dairy-free chocolate.

Making it lactose-free?
Make my quick, thick custard using lactose-free milk and a coconut whipping cream instead of double cream. Use lactose-free chocolate.

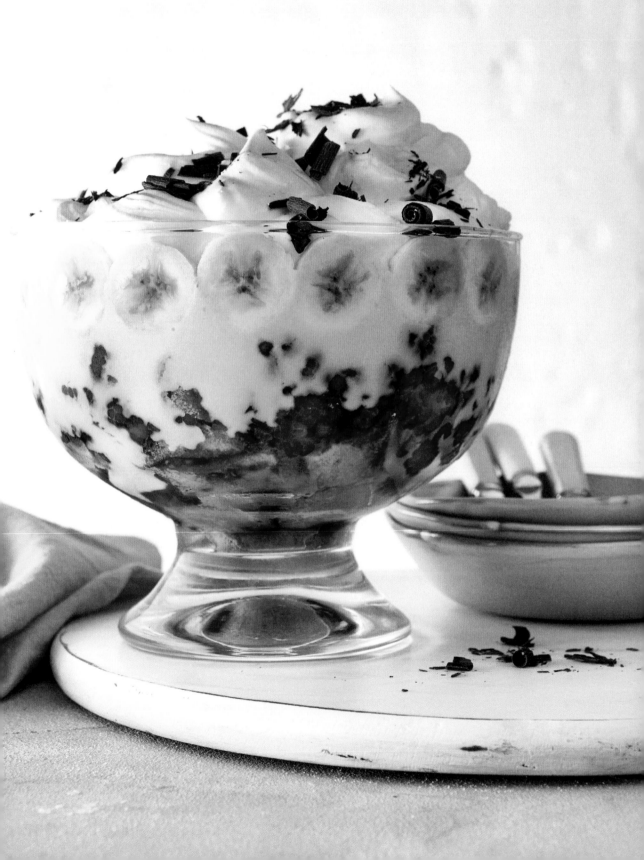

STICKY TOFFEE
Pudding

 low lactose — use lactose-free milk and cream

 vegetarian

 low fodmap — use lactose-free milk and cream

SERVES · 8

TAKES · 40 MINUTES

For the puddings

- 135ml / 9 tbsp milk
- 1 tbsp lemon juice
- 50g / 3½ tbsp butter, softened, plus extra for greasing
- 1 large egg
- 85g / 6 tbsp light brown sugar
- 110g / ¾ cup plus 1 tbsp gluten-free self-raising (self-rising) flour
- ½ tsp ground ginger
- ½ tsp bicarbonate of soda (baking soda)
- ¼ tsp gluten-free baking powder
- 1½ tbsp black treacle (molasses)

For the sticky toffee sauce

- 115g / generous ½ cup light brown sugar
- 1 tbsp black treacle (molasses)
- 275ml / generous 1 cup double (heavy) cream
- 90g / ⅖ cup butter

Nobody should have to miss out when it comes to dessert, especially not when sticky toffee pudding is on offer. The sponge is soft and light with a subtle caramel taste, which is perfect to soak up all that sweet, sticky sauce.

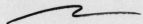

Preheat your oven to 160°C fan / 180°C / 350°F. Grease 6-8 mini pudding moulds with a little butter. In a jug (pitcher), mix your milk and lemon juice and allow to stand for 10 minutes until it curdles a little.

In a large mixing bowl, add the remaining pudding ingredients and whisk together until thoroughly mixed (I use an electric hand whisk for this). Slowly add the milk in two stages, whisking in between additions until well combined.

Pour your mixture into a jug and evenly divide between your buttered pudding moulds, leaving a 1cm / ⅜in gap at the top of each. Place the moulds on a baking tray and transfer to the oven for around 20-22 minutes until golden.

While they're baking, make your sticky toffee sauce. In a small saucepan, add all the sauce ingredients and place over a low heat. Allow the sugar to dissolve and everything to melt down, stirring occasionally. Bring to the boil and stir for 2-3 minutes before removing from the heat. Allow to cool until the sauce reaches a lovely pourable and sticky consistency.

Remove your puddings from the oven and allow them to sit in their moulds for about 1 minute, then carefully invert them onto serving plates. Serve with your sticky toffee sauce poured all over them.

TIP:
Want to make one large sticky toffee pudding? Simply double the mixture, pour into a greased casserole dish and cook for 40 minutes.

Making it dairy-free?
Use a (hard) dairy-free alternative to butter, dairy-free milk and dairy-free cream.

Making it vegan?
Follow the advice to make this dairy-free and replace the egg with 3 tbsp aquafaba (whisked until frothy).

MICROWAVE
Golden Syrup
SPONGE PUDDING

use a hard dairy-free butter alternative and dairy-free milk

use lactose-free milk

SERVES · 4–5

TAKES · 15 MINUTES

- 125g / ½ cup plus 2 tbsp butter, softened, plus extra for greasing
- 125g / 1 cup minus 1 tbsp gluten-free self-raising (self-rising) flour
- 125g / ⅔ cup caster (superfine) sugar
- 2 eggs
- ½ tsp vanilla extract
- 1 tbsp milk
- 80g / ¼ cup golden syrup, plus extra to drizzle
- 2 tbsp lemon juice

With a beautifully light and fluffy steamed sponge, topped with all that sweet, sticky, buttery golden syrup, this is simplicity at its finest. This was Mark's dad's favourite for school dinner dessert and I can totally see why!

Lightly butter a large, 1.2l / 5-cup microwavable pudding basin.

In a large mixing bowl, place your butter, flour, sugar, eggs, vanilla and milk and mix together until combined.

Spoon the golden syrup and lemon juice into the bottom of the buttered pudding basin and mix together, then spoon the pudding mixture on top of the syrup. Cover securely with cling film (plastic wrap) and pierce the cling film with the tip of a sharp knife a few times.

Microwave on medium/high (around 600W) for 5 minutes. Don't worry if you see the pudding rising up as the cling film will hold it in place. Allow to cool for 5 minutes before carefully turning out onto a plate. If you see any holes in the top, your pudding just cooked a little bit faster than it should have, but it will still taste just as good!

Drizzle with extra golden syrup and serve up straight away with custard.

TIP:
You can make individual puddings by using smaller microwavable pudding dishes and cooking the puddings for slightly less time.

EGG CONVERSION GUIDE

Did you know that a large egg here in the UK is actually bigger than in the USA, Canada and Australia? Me neither! That's why I thought I'd pop in a handy egg conversion guide in the back of this book to help make things simple.

That way, when a recipe calls for a small, medium or large egg, you can use the table below to work out exactly what that means for you. I've used UK egg sizes in all my recipes, so just convert from there.

	UK	USA	Canada	Australia
Small	53g and under	42.5g / 1½oz	42g / 1½oz	N/A
Medium	53-63g	49.6g / 1¾oz	49g / 1¾oz	43g
Large	63-73g	56.7g / 2oz	56g / 2oz	52g
Extra large	73g and over	63.8g / 2¼oz	63g / 2¼oz	60g
Jumbo	N/A	70.9g / 2½oz	70g / 2½oz	68g

And just in case you're too lazy to look at anything presented in a table (like I am), here's your cheat sheet! Maybe we can call a meeting of all our world leaders and agree on a uniform egg size in future?

So when a recipe in this book calls for a **small egg**, you should use a:

USA: medium egg
Canada: medium egg
Australia: large egg

When a recipe in this book calls for a **medium egg**, you should use a:

USA: large egg
Canada: large egg
Australia: extra-large egg

When a recipe in this book calls for a **large egg**, you should use a:

USA: extra-large egg
Canada: extra-large egg.
Australia: jumbo egg

INDEX

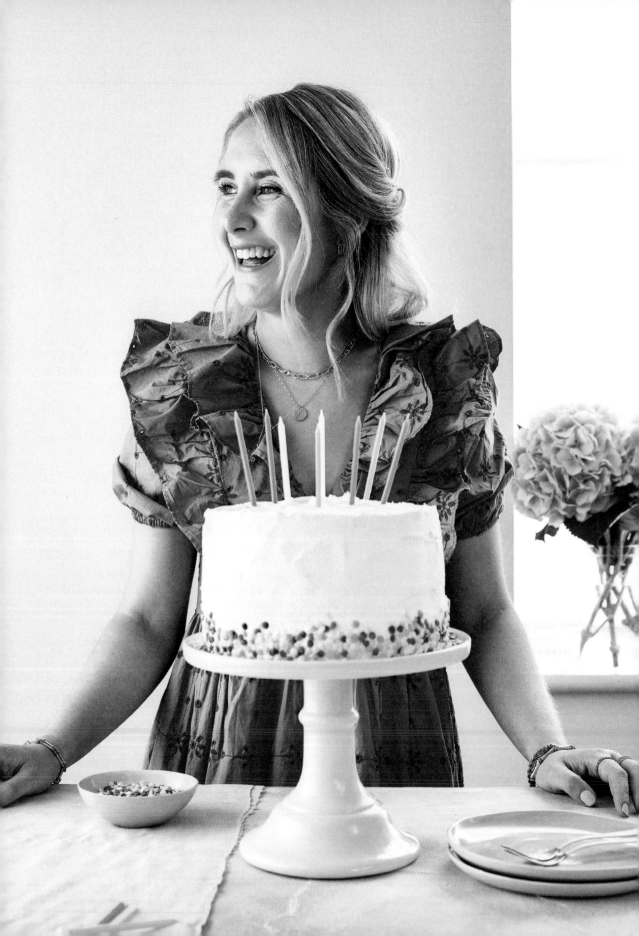

Thank you

Where on Earth do I start?!

It goes without saying that I want to extend a huge thank you to all the wonderful humans at Quadrille Publishing. Otherwise, this recipe book would still be just another idea floating around in my head.

I still struggle to process how this entire book was created from start to finish during a global pandemic, while putting the safety of everyone involved as priority. Yet, looking at the finished product, nobody would ever know, which says a lot about Quadrille. However, I do find it sad that I've only ever met most of you in person once, if at all! I'm very much looking forward to our next (socially distanced) meet-up (hopefully) very soon (if and when we're allowed).

First of all, I'm forever grateful to publishing director Sarah Lavelle, who believed in my idea enough to commission it. You totally understood the concept behind this book from day one in a way I never thought anyone would.

A billion thank yous to my editor, Harriet Webster - you are amazing at your job. I've never felt more confident doing something this big and scary because I know you're always there with all the answers! Thank you to copy editor Sally Somers for all your meticulous work and also for introducing me to the joys of a julienne peeler.

I'm not sure how Emily Lapworth did it, but she managed to read my mind, extract exactly how I wanted this book to be designed and improve upon it several million times. Thank you to your cat, Peach, for all her integral contributions during our online photoshoot sessions.

Thank you to Hannah Hughes for bringing this book to life with your mind-blowing photography and effortless vision. I think that by referring to each item of food as 'guys', my food photography has improved already.

I'm incredibly grateful for Emily Kydd, Alice Ostan, and Katy Gilhooly's magical food styling - you should all be accepted into Hogwarts for making my recipes look this good. Infinite high fives to Rebecca Newport for your beautiful crockery curation and all things prop styling throughout this book.

Thank you to Cat Parnell for your hair and make-up wizardry - because of you, I actually like how I look in a photo for the first time ever. Can you please follow me around and do this every day of my life?

Big thanks to what I call 'Team Laura' (Laura Willis and Laura Eldridge) and Ruth Tewkesbury for doing such an amazing job at shouting about this book and letting the world know that it exists.

I couldn't not thank my boyfriend, Mark, for being an infinitely level-headed, kind superhuman and my partner in crime. He's my trustworthy taste-tester who will always tell me whether my gluten-free recipes taste 'gluten-free' or not, with helpful critiques such as 'I'm 80% sure I'd eat this.' He contributed more recipes to this book than he wants to take credit for and without him, the fakeaways chapter in this book basically wouldn't exist. If it wasn't for his motivational speeches, I'd still be trying to write the first page of this book, curled up in a ball of stress with a peppermint tea that went cold several hours prior.

Thank you to my little dog, Peggy, who I can genuinely say has been my own personal cheerleader throughout writing this book. She never fails to put a smile on my face, no matter how I'm feeling.

You never say thank you to your mum and dad enough, so now I get to put it in writing! Thank you so much for always pushing me to be the best I can be, for supporting me through everything (the good and the not so good!) and for always understanding that my 'job' is a little unconventional and strange.

Thank you to my 'little' brother Charlie and his girlfriend Gemma for always eating/distributing (and hopefully enjoying?!) everything I bake. Please return all my plates and tupperware ASAP - this is your last warning.

A huge thank you to my hairdresser, Nikki, for fixing my hair (which had randomly turned blue during lockdown) just in time for the photoshoot for this book. And also for generally being an inspiring example of how to stay upbeat and strong, no matter what life throws your way.

I also have to thank my Ouma, Grandma, Grandad, Uncle Neil and Molly. Though none of you ever knew this book was going to exist, I know you would all have been super proud.

And finally, thank YOU for trusting me enough to spend your hard-earned money on this book. You seriously don't know how much that means to me - fingers crossed it was everything you were hoping for. I hope it reunites you with all the food you really miss and makes your gluten-free life that little bit easier.

Publishing Director
Sarah Lavelle

Junior Commissioning Editor
Harriet Webster

Copy Editor
Sally Somers

Art Direction and Design
Emily Lapworth

Photographer
Hannah Hughes

Food Stylist
Emily Kydd

Prop Stylist
Rebecca Newport

Make-up Artist
Cat Parnell

Head of Production
Stephen Lang

Senior Production Controller
Katie Jarvis

FSC
www.fsc.org
MIX
Paper from
responsible sources
FSC® C004592

First published in 2021 by Quadrille, an imprint of Hardie Grant Publishing

Quadrille
52–54 Southwark Street
London SE1 1UN
quadrille.com

Text © Becky Excell 2021
Photography © Hannah Hughes 2021
Design and layout © Quadrille 2021

All rights reserved. No part of the book may be reproduced, stored in a retrieval system, or transmitted in any form or by any means, electronic, electrostatic, magnetic tape, mechanical, photocopying, recording or otherwise, without the prior permission in writing of the publisher.

The rights of Becky Excell to be identified as the author of this work have been asserted by her in accordance with the Copyright, Design and Patents Act 1988.

Cataloguing in Publication Data: a catalogue record for this book is available from the British Library.

Reprinted in 2021 (four times)
10 9 8 7 6 5

ISBN: 978 1 78713 661 8

Printed and bound in Germany by Firmengruppe Appl, aprinta druck, Wemding

This book is not intended as a substitute for genuine medical advice. The reader should consult a medical professional in matters relating to their health, particularly with regard to symptoms of IBS and coeliac disease.

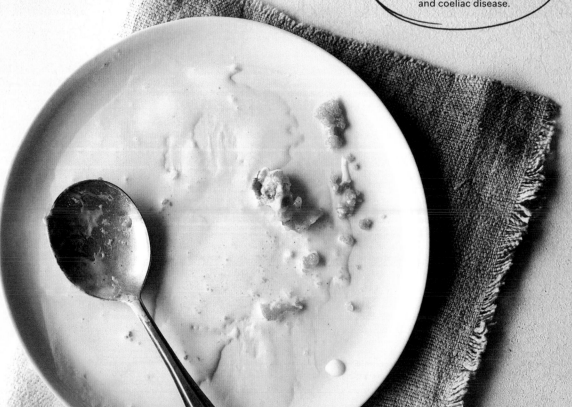

BECKY EXCELL is a full-time gluten-free food writer with a following of over 300,000 on her social media channels and 1 million monthly views on her award-winning blog. She's been eating gluten-free for over 10 years and has written recipes for numerous online publications, as well as doing cooking demos at events including the Cake and Bake Show. She gave up a career working in PR and marketing to focus on food full-time, with an aim to develop recipes which reunite her and her followers with the foods they can no longer eat. She lives in Essex, UK.

I CAN HAVE EVERYTHING…
you magically removed gluten-free stigma and told us that we can have everything… love you Becky!

Aisha

After getting my coeliac diagnosis I was completely lost but after finding Becky I found my confidence again and realised that I could make absolutely anything! **YOU HAVE SAVED ME.** Thank you xx

Laura

Becky's recipes have helped my 8-year-old since his coeliac diagnosis. He has been a keen chef for years but we've had to adapt quickly to gluten-free cooking and her recipes have played a large part in that. During lockdown, cooking played a large part in **CREATING A HAPPY PLACE** for us in the kitchen where he could create. He baked for all of our neighbours, delivering treats to their doorsteps, and they **DIDN'T GUESS FOR A SECOND THAT THEY WERE EATING GLUTEN-FREE.**

Debbie

The recipes make me feel like **I HAVE CHOICES AGAIN.** Things I haven't had for years I can now make! I don't have to miss out anymore which feels incredible! Thank you, Becky.

Ceri

ABSOLUTELY INSPIRATIONAL.
Becky's recipes are mouth-watering and allow for even the least creative cooks to make delicious gluten-free treats.

Candice

Your recipes have given me the confidence to bake, now my **WHOLE FAMILY ENJOYS THEM!**

Helen

Fantastic recipes and the detailed step-by-step guide for each recipe means they turn out perfect every time. **I NO LONGER FEEL LIKE I'M MISSING OUT.** Thanks Becky !

Bindu

YOU HAVE FOUND THE BAKER IN ME that I never knew existed. Me and my "gluten eating" family are forever grateful. Thank you Becky x

Hayley

Life after coeliac diagnosis has changed our lives but Becky's amazing foolproof recipes **BROUGHT US BACK TO WHAT NORMALITY USED TO BE!**

Crissie